WEIGHT LOSS SUCCESS

How I Lost 80 lbs With Intermittent Fasting And A Low Carb Diet

By Wendy Nicholson

Second Edition (black and white)

Editing and cover design: Sarah Nicholson
Photography and illustration credits: Canva.com and the Nicholson family album

ISBN (colour paperback print book) 9798405223742
ISBN (colour hardcover print book) 9798404503258
ISBN (black and white paperback print book) 9798746813428

DEDICATION

To all of you who have been on the yo-yo dieting roller coaster ride and are ready to change your future and find weight loss success. You can do it!

BEFORE
210 lbs

AFTER
130 lbs

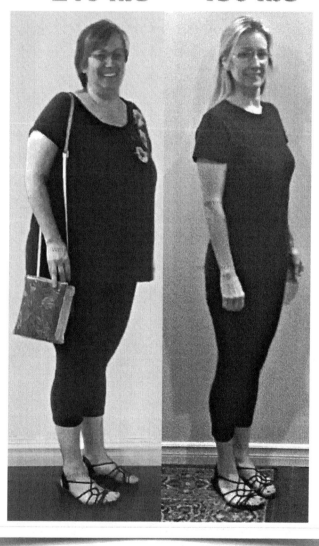

ACKNOWLEDGMENTS

I want to thank my 3 children for always encouraging me, for challenging me to question my comfort zones, and make me want to live a long and happy life.

Thanks to all the people who have been a part of my weight loss journey over the years through weight loss groups, walking buddies, etc. The online Facebook groups have been tremendous as well.

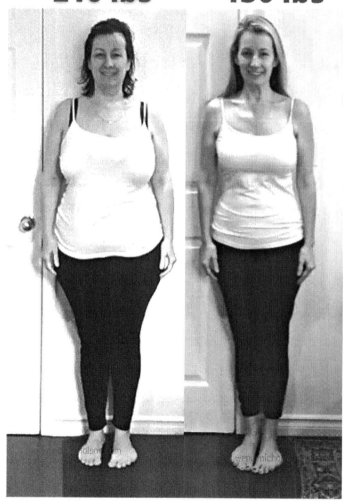

BEFORE
210 lbs

AFTER
130 lbs

CONTENTS

Before   After

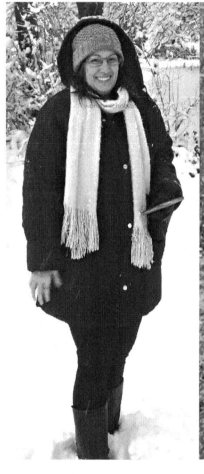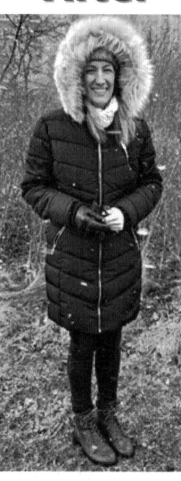

PREFACE

People have been asking me how I lost weight and got healthier. Well here it is! I documented my story and results in this book so now I could share it with you.

Weight loss is possible, even after age 50!

Here is a partial list of what's covered in this book:

WHAT MOTIVATED ME TO START LOSING WEIGHT

- High blood pressure
- High cholesterol
- Diverticulitis flare-ups
- Lethargy and fatigue
- Depression and moodiness
- Wanting to be active and do sports with family and friends
- Shop at "average-sized" clothing stores again…plus, many other factors.

WHAT MADE THE DIFFERENCE

- Admitting I am a carb-addict
- Daily habit changes
- A large online support group
- Watching videos by doctors and therapists
- Listening to podcasts
- Reading blogs and scientific research studies
- Encouragement from family and friends
- Focusing on my desire to not let my health keep deteriorating as I age (if I can help it!)

WHAT I CHANGED

- Started intermittent fasting
- Eating low-carb diets
- Taking out 95% of the processed foods and carbs (grains, sugars, etc.) from my regular diet
- Eating a large variety of meats and vegetables
- Cooking from scratch
- Cutting out fried fast foods/frozen foods
- Eating less fruits, dairy and nuts
- Drinking 0-carb drinks
- Emptying the fridge, freezer, and cupboards of all my "risky" foods

This book is made up of 21 Chapters. The headings are based on questions that you may have as you start on your own weight loss journey.

Also, you will find many recommended videos, lectures, and podcasts within the chapters.

These will give some of the background for what I learned and related to the topics in the chapters. There are some definitions for medical terms as well.

At the end of the book, you will see a reference list so you can do more research yourself.

I hope by reading my story, you can be inspired in your own journey towards improved health and weight loss success.

Here's to a brighter tomorrow!

DISCLAIMERS

1.

I am not a doctor. Any medical, health, diet or fitness information in this book is for educational and informational purposes only and is not to be used or relied on for any diagnostic or treatment purposes. This information should not be used as a substitute for professional diagnosis and treatment.

2.

Please consult your health care provider before making any health care decisions or for guidance about a specific medical condition. I expressly disclaim responsibility for any damages, loss, injury, or liability whatsoever suffered as a result of your reliance on the information contained in this book. Please note that this is NOT medical advice. Please do your own research.

3.

Regarding my background, these are my memories and opinions of my past. It is not my intention to defame or embarrass anyone. I am telling my story and my background to give some context into my experience with yo-yo dieting and my personal carb addiction.

4.

I am not connected to the doctors and professionals mentioned in this book and I only recommend them for educational and informational resources. I also do not agree with everything they recommend and do not currently endorse them for economic or marketing purposes.

5.

This book does not constitute medical advice, other than where specific doctors have been quoted and cited. Please consult a medical or health professional before you begin any weight loss program. There may be risks associated with intermittent fasting, LCHF, the Keto, AIP or any other diet mentioned in this book.

6.

By choosing to follow any of the information within this book, you assume all risks associated with those activities. Specific results mentioned in this book are not "typical" because every individual is different.

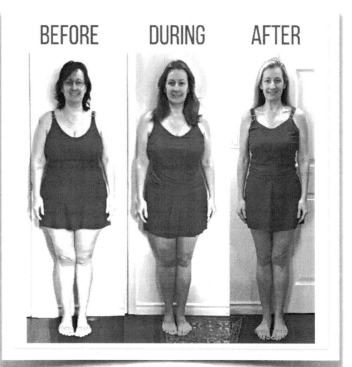

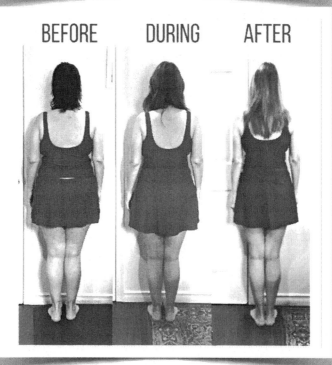

INTRODUCTION

Are you a "yo-yo dieter"?

Are you not sure if it's worth your time to try another diet?

If you answered yes, then you've been exactly where I have been.

After reading this book, you will find out which diet(s) worked for me and how I was able to start my recovery journey after being a "carb-aholic" for over 50 years.

If you suspect that you too are a carb-addict like me and you are ready to learn new things and get to the root of your carb addiction, then keep reading!

People have many reasons why they want to lose weight. Consider some of these reasons why:

* Wanting to be healthy for family and kids
* Helping to overcome binge eating and emotional eating
* Dealing with health concerns and multiple medications
* Increasing longevity
* Increasing mobility as we age
* Lessening health scares
* Helping with mood swings

What are a few of the top frustrations that dieters have?

- Diets have a 95% fail rate
- Eating healthy is expensive
- Weight loss is hard work

The truth is the path to success wasn't easy for me. I'm not going to sugar coat it, pun intended!

However, my ultimate goal was attained, and I even surpassed my own expectations!

After being tired of being obese, I found a solution that worked for me, and I achieved great results such as:

- Fitting into smaller clothes (size medium and small)
- Sharing clothes with my daughters
- Fewer wrinkles
- Less inflammation
- Having normal blood pressure
- Having a resting heart rate in a normal range
- Not having diverticulitis flare-ups
- Having more energy
- Being able to keep my balance if I trip
- Going to the gym and feeling "normal" in gym cloths
- Looking and feeling younger
- Improved moods

What about the costs?

I'm sure you have seen the price of health food or organic food at the grocery store. It seems very overpriced, right?

What if you could be on a diet that actually was less expensive each month than the way you are eating right now?

Well, I discovered that eating low carb was cheaper…after losing 80 lbs I am not needing to buy so many groceries!

So, keep reading…you will see how I found freedom from carb addiction, emotional eating and now feel empowered by taking back my health!

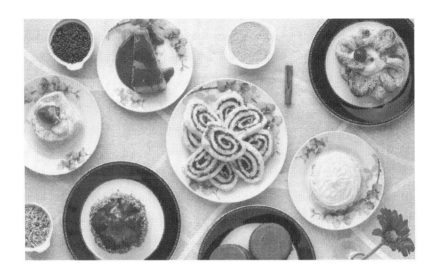

1 - SWEET TOOTH

WHEN DID YOU FIRST HAVE A SWEET TOOTH?

From as far back as I can remember, I had a "sweet tooth". I snacked when I was bored or angry. I would binge-eat cookie dough in secret at age 12.

Unfortunately, I became a binge eater with anorexic behaviours as well (*see more on the topic of eating disorders in Chapter 3*).

I hated overeating because I felt awful afterwards. But while I was overeating, the taste of sugar, bread, cookies, desserts, and fruit was enjoyable and energizing!

These were comfort foods for me. Yet, the more I ate, the more I craved. My "comfort" only lasted while I was eating.

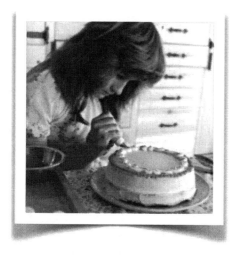

I took a cake decorating course around age 12, and over the years, would decorate cakes for family members and friends.

This made me feel fulfilled in that I could use my creative skills but also make other people like me with what I created for them. Early on, I was a people pleaser, and this became an easy way to make people happy.

I loved to bake since this would be rewarding…getting praise from others who enjoyed eating what I made.

In high school, I worked at a cake decoration and party supply store, so was around sweet foods a lot.

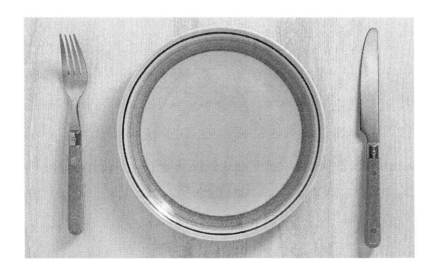

WHAT ARE FOOD TRAUMAS?

My earliest memories involved food and the trauma around food; what to eat, when to eat, and how much to eat…food was extremely regulated.

I was physically punished if I didn't eat the correct amount of food or types of food.

There are many of you who may have also been part of the "clean your plate club," with strict rules from family members about finishing everything that was served.

Sadly, I was taught to clean my plate instead of listening to my body's natural built-in way of letting me know when I was full.

Why was I supposed to clean my plate?

Firstly, my grandmother would tell me that leaving any morsel or scrap would worsen the plights of starving children in a far-off country.

And secondly, somehow, I would bring shame upon the family name if I left any food on my plate when I was at someone else's house.

I used to hold my nose while I tried to eat onions, bananas, mushrooms, etc. so that I wouldn't taste the food. I hated the texture of certain foods.

Feeling ashamed and afraid of being punished, I would try to force myself to eat. This would make me gag and even throw up, which was traumatic.

I will not forget being in first grade and hating my lunch since it would make me nauseated.

I threw it away in the garbage at school, but I got caught and was physically punished by my parents for that act of rebellion.

My family was obsessed with food because it was a huge part of our life on a homestead.

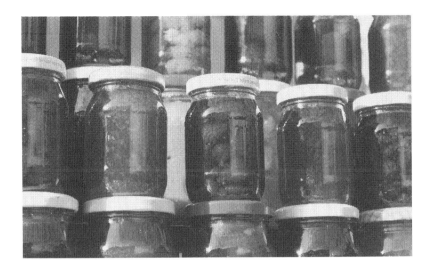

Growing up, we focused on:

- Growing a garden
- Harvesting the crops
- Preserving the food for the winter
- Cooking food from scratch

Traditionally, our main meals always contained a carb such as:

- Potatoes
- Rice
- Pasta
- Bread/buns

And every breakfast involved some form of carbs and sugar:

- Granola with honey
- Home-preserved fruit with syrup
- Pancakes/crepes
- French toast
- Waffles
- Cottage cheesecake
- Muffins
- Coffee cake
- Toast
- Cinnamon buns

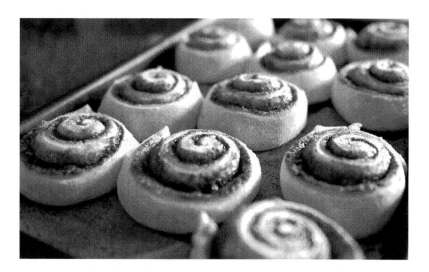

Meat was less important than the carbs. Yes, there were vegetables and salads, but they did not make up the bulk of the food we ate.

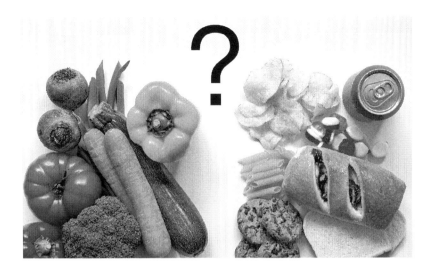

Some suppers were literally a freshly baked loaf of whole wheat bread in the middle of the table. That was it!

As well, every Sunday evening, we continued the multi-generational tradition of popcorn as the main meal. I continued that custom for years with my own kids as well.

WHAT FOODS WERE GOOD AND BAD?

When I was in grade school, I would trade my "good" food (an apple) for "bad" food (dessert cherry bars) with a friend on the school bus.

I craved "bad" foods like store bought white bread and processed cheese spread and would get excited if I got to go to a friend's house and have some of those taboo foods.

I also spent all my allowance on candy and chocolate bars.

Even though white bread and processed foods were seen as "bad", sugar was not seen in this way.

Both sets of my grandparents influenced me around food. When we would visit my grandparents in the U.S., my paternal grandfather cooked large meals full of carbs.

He also "spoiled" my brother and I by allowing us to buy as much candy as we wanted.

Although there were a lot of off-limit foods and substances when I was growing up, such as alcohol and drugs, sugar was not a taboo.

Growing up during the 70's and 80's, people who overate sugar were not seen as being addicted to a substance in the same way as those that were addicted to smoking, for example.

However, the substance addiction of sugar was very real and yet I never knew I was an addict until age 51!

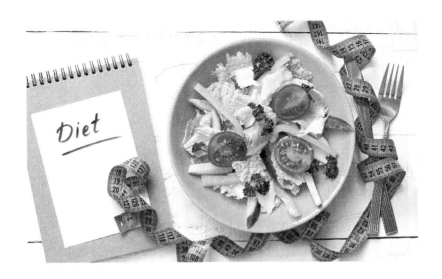

2 - DIETING BEHAVIOURS

WHEN DID YOU GO ON YOUR FIRST DIET?

I remember my 60-year-old grandpa being on the *Fit For Life* [19] diet and he had two rules about food:

- Only fruit before lunch
- No complex carbs eaten together

Since puberty, I was always dieting. In high school, I spent a large amount of my income from my part-time jobs on candy, soda, and chocolate bars.

During my teen years, I used to blame myself for being one of the "heaviest" girls in my class (no one was obese in my high school, back in the 80's). This shame led me to decades of dieting.

The most I weighed was 150 lbs in my teen years, which felt obese to me.

It was disheartening and discouraging. I was obsessed about my appearance and covering up my fat body. Since I sewed almost all my own clothes, I could make the clothes fit me depending on if I was losing or gaining weight.

Two of the diets that I remember the most were eating only salads for 14 days, and a water-fast for 5 days (my first "taste" of extended fasting).

Sure, I lost weight during these extreme elimination diets, but then I would gain it all back in a short amount of time.

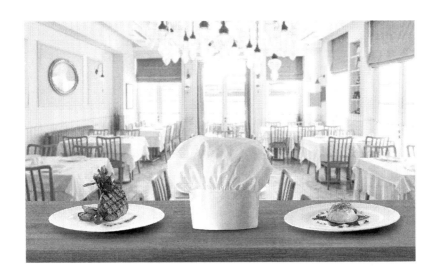

WHY PURSUE COOKING AS A PROFESSION?

After high school, I was encouraged to go to professional cooks training at college so I would be a better wife..."The way to a man's heart is through his stomach", I was told repeatedly.

During the first semester, I gained 30 lbs since I was around food all day long.

I worked at a restaurant after the first year of college but hated being seen as a second-class citizen...at this family restaurant, the cooks were not allowed to be seen by the customers.

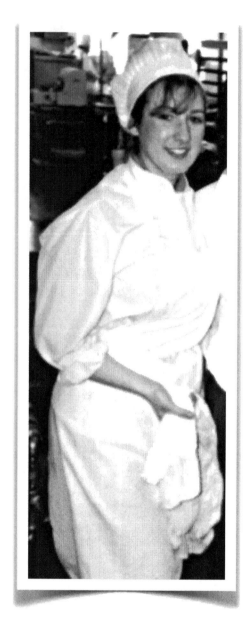

It was hard work in a small kitchen, and it made me choose a different career path.

I was glad in many ways to not be around food all day and this helped me to stop gaining the weight, for awhile.

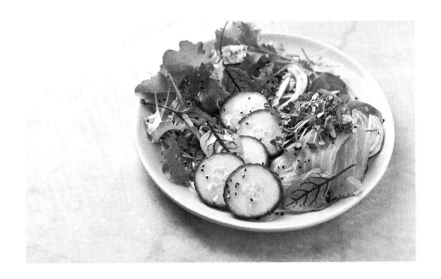

How many diets have you been on?

I would go on a diet, lose weight and people would notice and ask me what the secret was. Then I would informally coach others to try to lose weight too.

But I always gained the weight back.

I helped start and facilitate multiple small weight loss groups in Canada and Brazil in my 20's, 30's and early 40's.

Some weight loss groups I would start with a handful of women, others I joined, like Weight Watchers [28].

Most were religious based, bringing Bible verses and prayer into the mix.

A few of the diets I tried included:

* Fit For Life [19]
* Weigh Down Diet [17]
* Atkins [16]
* Paleo [24]
* AIP [27]
* Weight Watchers [28]

Other things I tried included meal replacement drinks and smoothies, diet pills, and numerous combinations of diets… anything to try to get smaller.

In my early 40's, when I lost 25 lbs on the Paleo diet, I offered a presentation at a "lunch and learn" at the government office where I worked.

Then, I hosted a weigh-in once a week for some of my co-workers to get together and see how much they had lost.

Of course, like all diets, they work 100% of the time at the beginning.

But for me, they also failed 100% of the time after several days, weeks or months.

The pitfalls and mistakes I found from most diets included:

* Time consuming (going to weekly meetings, month after month, year after year)
* Expensive (shakes, powders, pills, memberships)
* Tedious (counting calories or points)

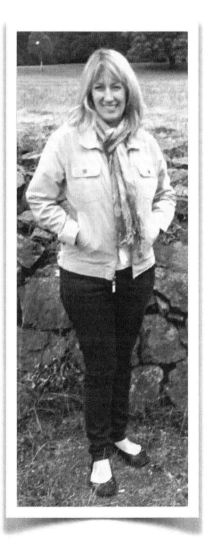

Some people have tried these diets and weight loss supplements and have found permanent weigh loss…they count in the 5%.

Unfortunately, I was one of the 95%. It was so frustrating to try diet after diet and not achieve lasting results.

So, after yo-yo dieting till my mid-40's, I was frustrated, confused, and was having health issues, as I will talk about in later chapters.

Finally, I found out that I had an eating disorder (actually several of them).

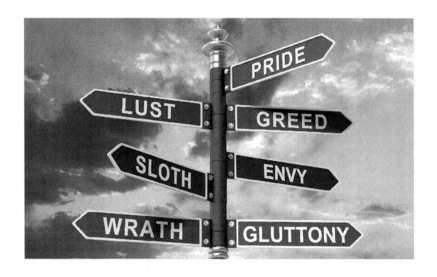

How do Religion and Culture Play a Role in Diet?

Most religions have customs and rules around food. Some have boundaries about what types of food to eat at which holidays. Some are vegetarian and others do extended fasts.

Overall, there are many religions and cultures that assume an overweight or obese person is a glutton and is "living in sin". And Gluttony was one of the "seven deadly sins".

However, putting this moral label on it ignores the reason behind why they are overweight or obese.

For myself, I grew up in a strictly religious culture with traditions around food. The religion was conservative

Evangelical Christianity and even though fasting was not a part of our religious customs, potluck suppers were.

There was a lot of emphasis on body image in our religion. Being thin was important to not be seen as a glutton or be seen as not being attractive.

When my first husband and I became evangelical overseas missionaries, we needed to speak in front of churches in order to fundraise for our salary.

This did put pressure on us to look a certain way. I know this helped keep me on the yo-yo dieting track so as to not be too overweight.

I remember hearing how a wife should stay thin and pretty in order to not make her husband be tempted to cheat with other women. The pastor had Bible verses to back this up. This put a lot of pressure on me!

Going on diets was seen as a way to dedicate myself to God's work of being the best Christian wife I could be.

One of the diets I went on while I was in Brazil was called the Weigh Down Workshop. [17]

We were told that God would help us lose the weight if we prayed all the time…sort of similar to the idea of "what would Jesus do"…what would Jesus want me to eat today?

Along with a few other co-workers, we all lost weight but none of us were able to keep it off after our small group dispersed.

It worked as long as we were meeting each week and watching the videos together.

I have since left the religion and am trying to look back and see where those body perfection issues came from and why they might still cause me to feel shame around my body.

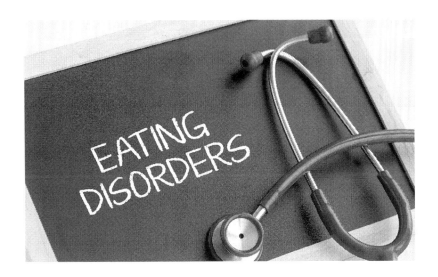

3 - EATING DISORDERS

WHAT WERE SOME OF YOUR EATING DISORDERS?

My journey into discovering my own eating disorders began in the fall of 2017, when I was dealing with a difficult situation in my life and family.

While I was waiting to see a therapist in-person, I thought I would look for therapists online and I stumbled upon someone who specialized in eating disorders.

When looking at my own food trauma symptoms, I started looking into eating and trauma.

I watched YouTube videos by Kati Morton, listened to podcasts and uncovered the fact that I had several eating disorders that I didn't even know existed.

But their description fit my symptoms and I was thrilled to know that I wasn't the only one dealing with these issues.

RECOMMENDED

"Eating disorders explained: Anorexia, bulimia, Ednos binge" playlist from the **Kati Morton** YouTube channel. [46]

I now can admit that I have varying degrees of 4 types of eating disorders that can all be traced back to before I went through puberty:

- Orthorexia [25]
- Avoidant/Restrictive Food Intake Disorder (ARFID) [36]
- Anorexia nervosa [20]
- Binge eating [46]

There is a 5th type of eating disorder called Bulimia. [3] Most people know Bulimia as the one where people will force themselves to throw up after they eat something, which leads to becoming malnourished. There is also a version of this with fitness and working out known as Exercise Bulimia.

I never did make myself throw up to lose weight. I sometimes would overexercise to try to lose weight, but that was rare.

With so much attention given to food in my family-of-origin, Orthorexia was actually enforced and encouraged. There is a list of warning signs and symptoms from the National Eating Disorders website which helps to define it: [25]

DEFINITIONS

"Orthorexia
- *Compulsive checking of ingredient lists and nutritional labels*
- *An increase in concern about the health of ingredients*
- *Cutting out an increasing number of food groups (all sugar, all carbs, all dairy, all meat, all*
-    *animal products)*
- *An inability to eat anything but a narrow group of foods that are deemed 'healthy' or 'pure'*
- *Unusual interest in the health of what others are eating*
- *Spending hours per day thinking about what food might be served at upcoming events*
- *Showing high levels of distress when 'safe' or 'healthy' foods aren't available*
- *Body image concerns may or may not be present"* [25]

Related to Avoidant/Restrictive Food Intake Disorder (ARFID), all my childhood trauma around being forced to eat foods I didn't like made me feel guilty for not eating certain foods...for being a "picky eater".

DEFINITIONS

"Avoidant/Restrictive Eating Disorder (ARFID) is an eating disorder like no other. The physiological constriction of the mouth tissues, throat, and digestive tract from the fear stops the ability to eat a variety of foods. Malnutrition from ARFID causes many medical issues, including fatigue and loss of motivation. Because ARFID is a sensory disorder as well as an eating disorder, its cure is through somatic treatment." [36]

Now that I was learning about eating disorders and that I had ARFID, it was so liberating.

Throughout my life, I have had a heightened sense of taste and smell, as anyone who has lived with me can attest to.

It has affected me in various ways, including becoming malnourished if I was on diets for too long.

Over the years, I have tried to learn to eat the foods I used to gag on when I was young and have had moderate success so far.

By changing my environments and habits, I have been able to keep functioning and not let this cripple or affect me daily.

Even though I have this trauma from my past (which is not fun to live with), I can learn from it and move on and find new habits to help me exist in society.

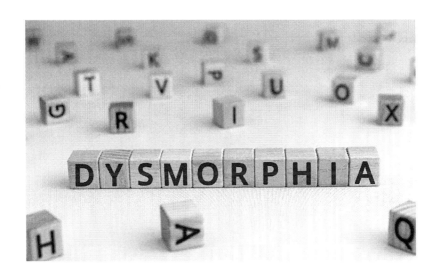

4 - BODY DYSMORPHIA

WHAT IS BODY DYSMORPHIA?

DEFINITIONS

"Body dysmorphic disorder is a mental health disorder in which you can't stop thinking about one or more perceived defects or flaws in your appearance — a flaw that appears minor or can't be seen by others. But you may feel so embarrassed, ashamed, and anxious that you may avoid many social situations." [2]

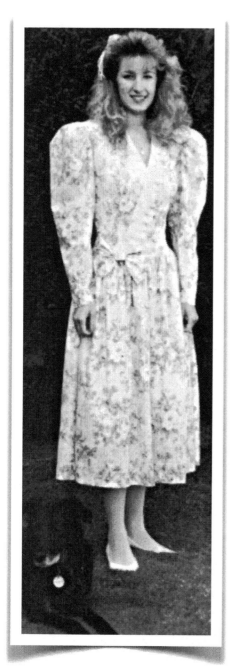

I always felt fat and hated my body and cannot remember a time that I didn't feel fat...even when I was an "average" weight of 130 lbs.

Later, I learned this is called body dysmorphia.

No matter my actual size, there was always a disconnect with how much I weighed and what I thought I looked like.

When I look at photos from the past, it is unfathomable to me that I was as slim as the picture shows.

It feels distorted...like looking at someone else.

Looking back, there seems to be at least 3 factors that led to this including:

1. Being raised in a legalistic, strict home

2. Enforced modesty by the conservative religion I was raised in

3. Being a woman in a society that often treats women as objects, and if they are not beautiful enough, they are invisible and ignored (so, if I was ignored, then I must not be thin and pretty)

As an adult, I can see there were life events that took place that made me gain weight or go on diets.

These major changes to my living situations caused fluctuations in my eating and my body that further stressed my body image issues:

* Moving and travelling a lot
* Living in Canada, US, and Brazil
* Giving birth to 3 children
* Breastfeeding
* Stresses from 2 marriages

These events would derail my diets or else motivate me to lose weight again.

For a short time, I weighted 115 lbs when I was 29 (and after having 3 babies and living in Brazil).

The heaviest I weighed was 165 lbs, even during my 3 pregnancies but, in my mind, I felt like I was 200 lbs.

I never weighed the same for any 12-month period…always up and down by 15-30 lbs each year so I always had a range of clothing sizes in my closet.

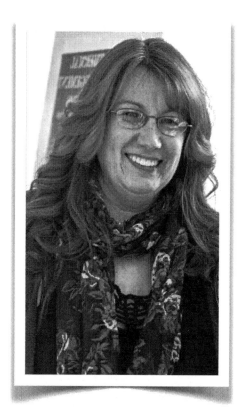

Then, in my late 40's when I did tip the scales at the 200 lbs mark, I finally understood how much body dysmorphia I had dealt with all those years.

Once I was obese, I literally had nothing to wear.

It was strange to take all my pants, jeans, and button-up shirts to the second-hand store.

I started to only wear black leggings and baggy tops.

I had become one of "those" people, wearing "fat clothes".

With so many changes to my wardrobe, I finally started to realize how messed up my brain had been, now that the clothes were matching what my brain had told me for decades…I WAS FAT!

Now, I will say here that I know some people have been in the overweight or obese category from a younger age than me.

And, when I started to actually live life in a larger body, I could see things from a whole new perspective.

There were new challenges I faced which I had not actually faced previously.

I could empathize for everyone who struggled with body issues and eating disorders as I had and this time it was obvious, not just all in my head!

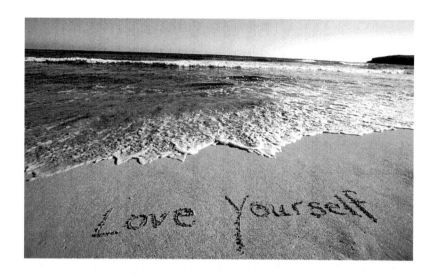

WHAT DOES BODY POSITIVE MEAN?

In writing this, I am not wanting to shame or judge anybody else.

I am sharing my experiences and what I have learned by being on all sides…an advocate for diets, then an anti-diet advocate, and back to finding a solution to the issue.

It is only recently that there has been greater acceptance of bodies that are bigger, and I understand everybody is on their own journey.

With all the years of yo-yo dieting, and mostly staying under the "obese" category, I still had body dysmorphia. I still had the same body issues around modesty and trying to make sense of an aging body.

Over the years, I have seen therapists, dieticians, doctors, and listened to hundreds of hours of podcasts on topics about dieting and health.

Through all this research, I finally ran across the body positivity/anti-dieting movement.

In this movement, I learned terms such as "fat acceptance," "intuitive eating," "thin privilege", and messages about reverse shaming the "diet cultures." We were never allowed to use the words "fat" or "obese".

I also learned the serious health conditions from being overweight are often disregarded – even when they can be reversed when people lose the weight.

Looking for relief from the difficulty of my body issues, I had hoped that the body positivity mindset could be a solution.

But in the groups, we were not allowed to talk about diets, or healthy eating, or losing weight. We were encouraged to never step on the weigh scale again.

There seemed to be a disconnect from the mind and body.

Basically, it was about accepting everyone no matter their size, or health conditions, and ignoring that there were ways to get healthier. Later, I could see that anyone who talked about wanting to lose weight was shamed or silenced it seemed.

But at the time, it was very convincing for me when I was obese and just wanting to feel accepted and loved.

I don't believe most of the folks in that community know their message can have long-term detrimental impacts on people, including myself. I think most have good intentions.

So, I stopped stepping on the weight scale, stopped caring, and tried to "love" my body as the body positive groups told me I should. "Love yourself!" That is what I was told to do.

Eventually, I became disillusioned with the movement when I saw my health continually getting worse.

However, by listening to the activists, I postponed facing the growing number of health conditions I was developing by being obese.

Since I was mostly listening to one side of the story, I ignored the root cause of my issues. Personally, I feel I may never have developed diverticulitis if I had not bought into that message.

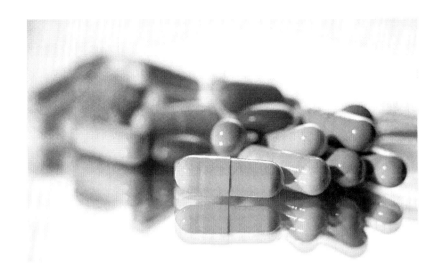

5 - HEALTH ISSUES

WHAT HEALTH ISSUES DID YOU HAVE FROM BEING OBESE?

I want to go back a few years and tell you a bit about my story related to health concerns in my earlier 40's.

- Life was stressful.
- My government job was stressful.
- My marriage was stressful.

I also had heart palpitations. I'd wake up in the middle of the night, gasping for air, with the sensation of an elephant on my chest.

I started to have thyroid problems and other autoimmune symptoms which included:

- Fatigue
- Joint pain
- Sensitivity to cold
- Mind fog
- Hair loss
- Shortness of breath

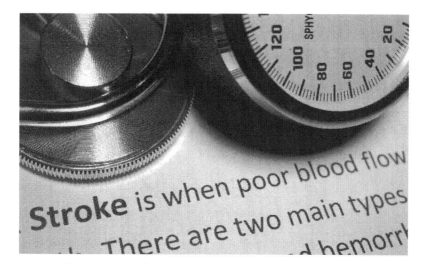

WHAT IS A TIA?

At the age of 43, I woke up one morning and couldn't walk very well. The right side of my body was weak.

My second husband, who had a masters in Neuroscience, could see right away that I had the signs of a stroke and he drove me to the hospital.

After multiple tests, the neurologist found that I had a small blood clot in my brain and had suffered a mini stroke, a transient ischemic attack (TIA). [33]

After more tests, including a "bubble test", they discovered I had a congenital heart defect called an atrial septal defect (ASD). [1]

DEFINITIONS

"An atrial septal defect (ASD) is a hole in the wall (septum) between the two upper chambers of your heart (atria). The condition is present at birth (congenital)." [1]

This shocked me since it was out of the blue and there was no family history of strokes.

Even though the neurologist said it was because of the ASD and bad luck, I started to suspect that I had become malnourished and that this may have contributed to the stroke.

The previous year I had started the Paleo diet. Due to my eating disorder and strong resistance to certain foods, the Paleo diet did not work well for me.

It called for us to eat organ meat, avocados, and many other foods. Due to my ARFID eating disorder, I hated these foods and so just couldn't tolerate them in my diet.

Though I had lost weight with this diet, it was becoming obvious that I was not getting a healthy amount of nutrition and this lasted for too long.

After my stroke, I slowly went off the Paleo diet and I started gaining weight again. I finally started to give up on trying to stay at a normal weight.

Up until age 47, I was only in the overweight category.

Then I became obese, and my BMI went above 30 (most doctors recommend a BMI of under 25 - see Chapter 14).

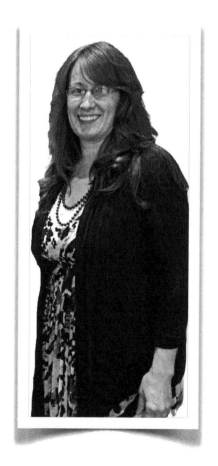

Realizing that I was more overweight than I had ever been, I didn't know what to expect.

Initially, I had fewer and fewer health issues, as I gained weight. It felt like I was no longer malnourished.

Maybe dieting had been the problem, I thought. So, for a short time, I was starting to feel better.

Here are 7 things that I noticed after I stopped dieting:

1. I didn't feel cold all the time
2. I didn't need the windows open to feel like I could breathe fresh air
3. I stopped getting frequent colds
4. My acne cleared up significantly
5. My hair was thicker
6. My nails weren't brittle
7. I had less insomnia

I felt better in the short term, but that did not last long.

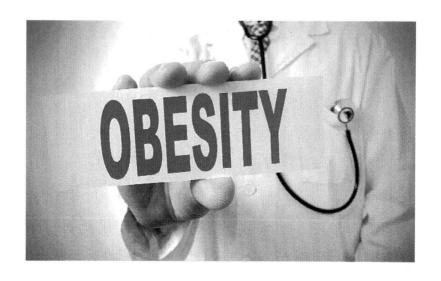

WHAT OTHER HEALTH PROBLEMS ARE RELATED TO OBESITY?

RECOMMENDED

"The Cancer Code with Dr. Jason Fung – Diet Doctor Podcast" from the **Diet Doctor** YouTube channel. [29]

After a couple of years being in the obese category, I started experiencing other health issues and ignored what my body was saying to me.

It was easier to assume it was "just life," that it was just what I had to live with. Or that it was just "this stage" in my life... perimenopause, etc.

I finally reached my heaviest weight of over 210 lbs, but I had stopped getting on the weigh-scale for a couple of years so I may have been over 210 lbs at some point.

With a BMI of over 35, I was wearing clothes at sizes XXL-XXXL and even plus size 1X and Size 20 pants.

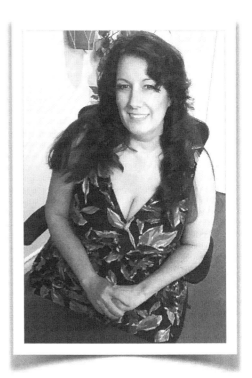

My bras were 42DD and 44E.

As I gained, weight I also developed several new health issues.

First, I developed high blood pressure, though I had never had an issue with this before, not even during my 3 pregnancies.

Second, I needed to start taking daily statin drugs for high cholesterol.

Third, I developed balance and flexibility issues. I broke my nose slipping on the ice one winter since I could not balance myself in my larger body.

Then, the following summer, I fell and broke my ankle, possibly due in part to my larger body size and not being in shape or flexible.

Lastly, I gained serious digestive issues. When I was 50, I was in the emergency room overnight with terrible stomach pains. I was diagnosed with diverticulitis. [22]

There was a risk I might need surgery for diverticulitis. This would involve a surgeon removing part of my colon. I was shocked and horrified to hear this!

In retrospect, it was the main catalyst to jolt me out of my haze, shine a light on the fact I had messed up my body, and show me that I needed to work at making it function well again.

In summary, from 2017 to 2020, I had new health issues that I had not had before I was obese.

These included:

- High blood pressure and high cholesterol
- Daily high resting heart rate (above 90 bpm)
- Diverticulitis and stomach polyps
- Fibroids
- Memory loss

Psychologically, being obese had taken its toll and impacted me in the following 3 ways:

1. Embarrassment and anxiety when exercising in public

2. Not being able to participate in activities I really enjoyed doing when I was in better shape such as swimming, going to the beach, riding my bike, and playing tennis

3. Feeling depressed about going clothes shopping and having nothing fit me

I hated my physical appearance, wanted to fade into obscurity and didn't like to get my picture taken.

Hiding behind people and objects in photographs became normal and I wore baggy black or patterned clothes to cover my big body.

Keeping my hair long made me feel I could draw attention away from my body.

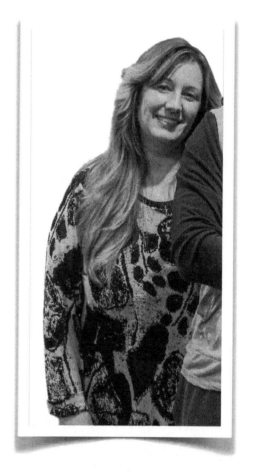

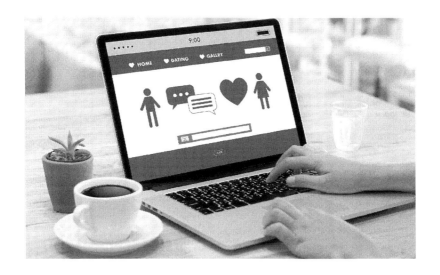

6 - ONLINE DATING

WHAT IS IT LIKE TO DATE WHILE BEING OVERWEIGHT?

After my second marriage ended in 2018, I came face to face with my body dysmorphia on a very personal level.

Initially, after the separation, I dealt with depression and was not motivated to take care of myself. I "let myself go" even more than I had in any previous years.

To be honest, I had to ask myself…did my 2nd marriage fail because I was obese?

Both my marriages were stressful but I had not been obese in my first 20-year marriage so I couldn't specifically pin-point that on being the main reason my 2nd one failed. It was only in the last year that I became obese.

I see now that my body dysmorphia impacted my attitudes about sex, self-image and confidence, all of which did play a role in both those relationships (hindsight is 20/20).

So, after 6 months of reflecting on my "failed" relationships, feeling lonely and depressed, I realized that I couldn't stay that way…I wanted to try to find love again.

As I joined several dating apps, I found some men accepted me at the weight I was at. It was an ego boost to find men who found me attractive and wanted to date me…I was not invisible after all!

Many men actually preferred a "voluptuous" or "curvy" woman!

There were other men though, that never responded, and one even messaged me to tell me that I was not his "type"! That hurt…and I knew what he meant.

So, I started going on dates and feeling excited that I could find some romance and be intimate again. I also learned to have sex with the lights on, as I got more comfortable in my body.

A few guys I dated had only been with slim women before me. Others did not want a long-term relationship once they saw I was not going to be into the same sports that they were into.

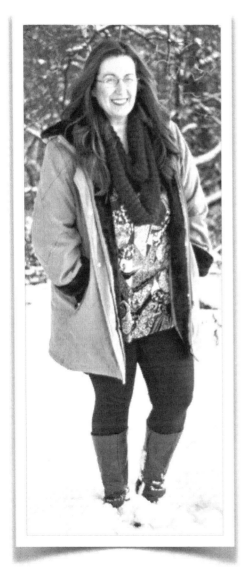

Those men were ultimately looking for a thin, "fit", athletic woman.

I had only one full-body picture on the online dating profiles, and I was wearing a winter coat and had a scarf on.

I remember wearing some type of scarf almost year round.

And of course, I had my long hair to help cover me.

There were no recent pictures of me wearing a bathing suit or even wearing jeans and a T-shirt. I didn't even own a pair of jeans anymore.

For the previous 3 years, I had only been wearing black leggings with elastic waist bands and baggy shirts.

I had taken all my thin clothes to the second-hand store and my bathing suit was a red "tankini" and looked more like a dress.

Originally when I started online dating, I was desperate to find a long-term relationship since I felt so lonely (after a combined 28 years between 2 marriages).

After one year and going on lots of dates, the Covid-19 pandemic hit in 2020.

This put a damper on my ability to find a deep connection and a long-term relationship. Online dating dramatically changed when the lockdown and stay-at-home orders were in place.

So, my desire to seek out another husband was lessening, and it was out of my control in many ways.

Accepting my responsibility for my past, current and future relationships and finding connection, partnership and love again was one of the catalysts for making me want to take better care of my body and health.

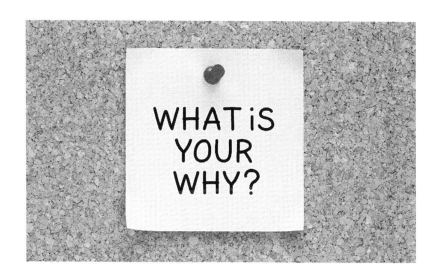

7 - MOTIVATIONS

WHAT MOTIVATES PEOPLE TO LOSE WEIGHT?

Have you daydreamed about having health and mobility as you got older?

That was me and I knew there just had to be a way that I could get healthier and lose the weight.

To deal with all the issues I listed in Chapter 5, I started on a path towards improved health. I started seeing a dietician, a doctor, and a psychiatrist in order to get help. Some of their advice was good, some not so good (*see Chapter 20*).

Slowly, I started losing weight by cutting down on portions, snacks and skipping a meal here and there. Or, I would stop eating breads for a week, for example.

I lost about 15 lbs in 2019 and another 15 lbs in 2020. But it was 3 steps forward and 2 steps back over that 2-year time frame.

Then, I turned 51 and decided enough was enough.

With the Covid-19 pandemic and the studies that showed that obese people faired much worse if they got the virus, it motivated me even more to change my habits and behaviours.

In January of 2021, I set a challenge of not going on another date with a guy until I was at my goal weight of 135 lbs.

That was one way to jump-start my weight loss!

Yes, it may sound fickle to have the goal of going on a date, but hey, we all need something to motivate us at times!!

Little did I know where my weight loss journey would take me…achieving and surpassing my original goal and having this story to tell!

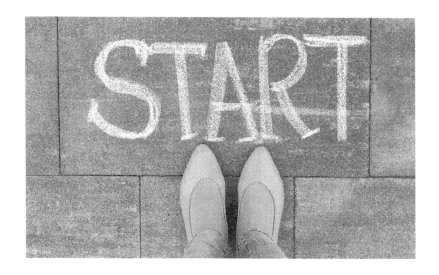

How do you get started?

I started researching, watching videos and lectures, reading blogs, and listening to podcasts. This is the steep part of the learning curve when we are learning something new. But it's also fun and exciting.

Being a very curious person, I put all my effort into this.

Having been on so many diets, I knew what calories were, but I didn't know much about carbs.

The more I learned about carbohydrates, the more I saw that I was a carbohydrate-addicted person. I started seeing things with new eyes.

It seemed as if our North American dietary culture was based on carbs!

This helped take some of the weight off my shoulders of feeling like it was all my fault that I was carb-obsessed and couldn't stop eating them.

I knew that if I continued to have an unhealthy relationship with carbs, I would be in trouble.

After starting to learn about the low carb and Keto diet combined with intermittent fasting, I started to implement what I was learning.

And I started to see results!

During the first month, I lost 14 lbs after being stalled at the same weight for the previous 6 months.

I found doctors and professionals online that seemed to make a lot of sense and had scientific research to back it up. They also combined thousands of anecdotal stories from their patients to reinforce what they had to say.

There were several Facebook groups I joined and I also signed up for an online paid membership site for a month.

Then I listened to some YouTube videos by Dr. Robert Cywes (he calls himself the "Carb Addiction Doc") and I saw a whole new perspective about carb addiction.

Now, as I learned more about carbs and what insulin does in our bodies, it was very eye opening to understand that carbs act like a drug.

I would go on Pinterest and find posts of people who had tackled their carb addiction and pinned posts related to intermittent fasting and low carb recipes.

In my search for resources, I also found there were other Facebook groups for women going through menopause and doing intermittent fasting.

I started to really listen to my body; what ached, what medical test results were concerning and how did I feel after I ate certain foods.

RECOMMENDED

"Sugar: The Bitter Truth" from the **University of California Television (UCTV)** YouTube channel. [35]

I had first watched Robert Lustig's video back in 2012, but I didn't really take it to heart. Then I had switched over to listening to the Paleo folks and followed that diet instead of looking at my carb addiction.

Here I was, 9 years later, finally addressing the carbs and sugar issue that had dominated so much of my life and failed dieting attempts.

Recognizing some days would be easier than others to tackle my 50+ year carb addiction helped me get over the beginning stages of this journey.

I needed to take baby steps, one day at a time.

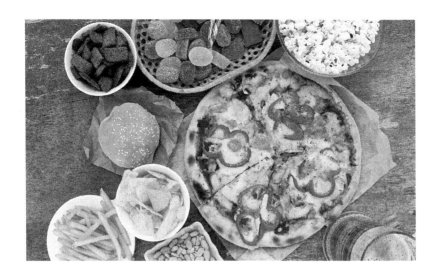

8 - CARBS AND SUGAR

WHAT IS THE SAD DIET?

Most people do not have a farm or even a vegetable garden to grow and raise their own food. Therefore, the foods we order at fast food restaurants and family restaurants and what we buy at the grocery store make up our diets.

The first time I heard about the Standard American Diet (SAD) [31] was when I was researching the Paleo diet back in 2012.

I learned that junk food, processed foods, soft drinks and fried foods all fall under the category of the SAD diet.

It made sense to call it "sad" as it was the root cause of the "sad" state of health and obesity issues that so many people deal with in North America.

The SAD diet refers to the traditional food pyramid that most of the US and Canada adhere to where they encourage carbs to be consumed more than any other food.

Like many people, it is the diet I was raised on.

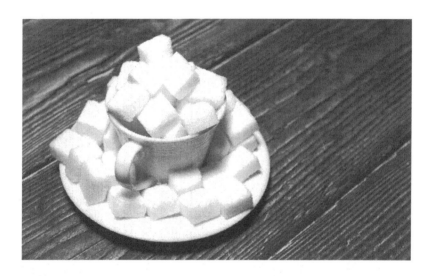

HOW MUCH SUGAR DO WE EAT?

In comparison to when I was growing up, I think more and more people are starting to get the picture that sugar is bad for our bodies.

But that does not stop the companies that earn money from sugary foods from continuing to market and sell us those foods.

For example, when we are at a check-out counter at the grocery store, there is a display stand with multiple types of candy and chocolate bars – and even sometimes a mini fridge with cold soft drinks.

Have you ever read the labels and been shocked like I was at how much sugar is in those candy bars and drinks?

RECOMMENDED

"Is Cancer Caused By Sugar?" from the **Mark Hyman, MD** YouTube channel. [38]

I saw a website where there were pictures of common foods and beverages alongside stacks of sugar cubes to represent how much sugar was in each food or drink.

This was sickening to see how much sugar I was consuming when I ate or drank these.

I did watch some videos by Gary Taubes as well over the past 10 years, but nothing really sunk in and made me change my habits until 2021.

RECOMMENDED

"Interview With Dr. Jason Fung and Gary Taubes." from the **CrossFit** YouTube channel. [5]

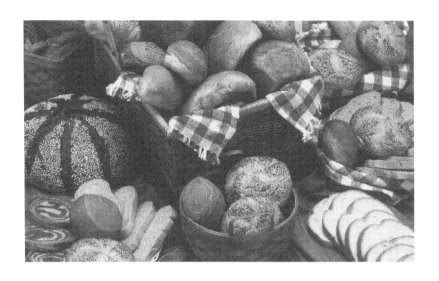

HOW ARE BREADS AND GRAINS SIMILAR TO CANDY?

RECOMMENDED

"*Wheat belly: Avoid these 7 common mistakes*" from the **Dr. Davis Infinite Health** YouTube channel. [37]

While we all may be gaining an understanding about the dangers of eating too much sugar, what is still not as well-known is how carbohydrate foods essentially turn into sugar in our bodies.

That piece of toast, cinnamon bun, tortilla, bowl of rice, or plate of pasta also turns into sugar when we digest it.

If you look at nutritional labels and look at the number associated with carbohydrates, it paints a very different picture than if we are only looking at calories.

Society is not helping those of us with a carb addiction…it is in fact trying to persuade us we need to snack on carbs "to keep our energy up."

All the marketing and advertising makes it hard to resist the tempting pictures and slogans of delicious looking carb foods.

In contrast, farmers don't have the money to advertise. Have you seen any advertisements for eating a salad every day? Have you ever watched a commercial for unprocessed vegetables?

When I really started to take my health seriously and learn that the bread and grains I ate were actually making me obese, it was like the light switch turned on in my brain!

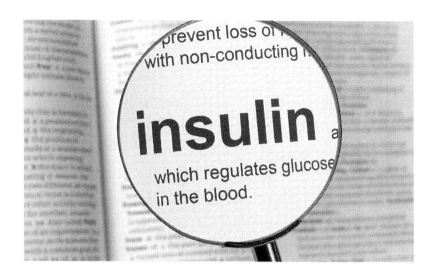

What is Insulin Resistance?

Dr. Fung uses the analogy of a fridge and freezer.

If we keep filling up the fridge with frequent meals, our body will only use that food up and the freezer will stay full (our stored fat).

If we stop filling up the fridge, then our bodies will start using up what is in the freezer.

The carbs I ate were all converted into sugar in my body. And anytime I ate more carbs, my body stored the sugar as fat, thanks to the hormone called insulin.

The only thing I knew up till that point about insulin was that people with Type 2 diabetes had to take it in order to regulate their blood sugar.

Once I started learning more about insulin and how every time I ate, I was raising my insulin levels, I could see the link between insulin and how our bodies could become "insulin resistant". [23]

DEFINITIONS

"Insulin and insulin resistance drive obesity. Refined carbohydrates such as white sugar and white flour cause the greatest increase in insulin. These foods are quite fattening. This does not mean that all carbohydrates are similarly bad. There is a substantial difference between 'good' carbohydrates (whole fruits and vegetables) and 'bad' (sugar and flour)." [30]

I first learned that most obese people are actually pre-diabetic while watching the video by Dr. Jason Fung.

If I was on the road to becoming a Type 2 diabetic, I better do something to change my ways!

I did not want to have to take insulin every day as a diabetic. Losing my eyesight or a limb due to Type 2 diabetes would be devastating.

RECOMMENDED

"Dr. Jason Fung - 'A New Paradigm of Insulin Resistance'" from the **Low Carb Down Under** YouTube channel. [13]

So, basically it came down to this…I was fat because I was eating too many carbs, too often.

The more carbs I ate, the more carbs I craved. But my body stopped me from overeating real food, so I never had to portion control.

I didn't overeat a steak, or eggs, or chicken, or salad, or vegetables. However, that natural limit is not there to protect me when I was eating foods that caused an insulin spike.

It was not me, or my lack of motivation to stop eating that piece of cake or brownie.

No! The carbs themselves were making me crave more carbs…like a drug!

If I never ate sugar, high carb, or processed foods, I wouldn't crave sugar, high carb, or processed foods.

It seemed simple enough.

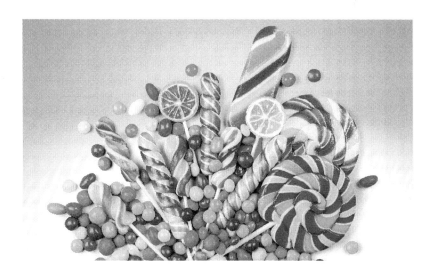

9 - CARB ADDICTION

WHY DO SOME PEOPLE NOT GAIN WEIGHT FROM CARBS?

For many reasons, some people don't gain weight when they eat carbs.

Genetics, family-of-origin history, environment, and habits are all reasons why some people (and even cultures) can eat carbs and not have the insulin resistance issue that causes obesity, diabetes, and more.

However, for people who are part of the societies where carbs are a large part of their diet, it seems many, like myself, do struggle with carb addiction.

We hear terms such as:

- Emotional eating
- Comfort foods
- Cheat meals
- Carb loading
- Snacks
- Happy hour

…and we all will think of foods and drinks that usually consist of carbs.

I even bought a cookbook once that was called *Comfort Foods* and sure enough, all the meals had some type of grains, starches or sugars in their recipes.

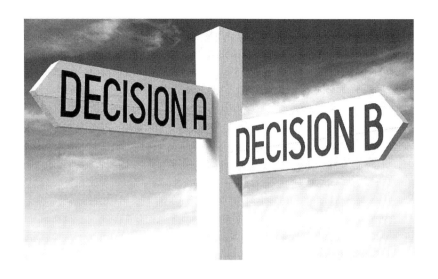

How is carb addiction like other addictions?

Many smokers quit and quit successfully. The same is true for some people who are addicted to other substances including alcohol and heroin.

However, when some quit one addiction, they may just transfer their substance of choice over to carbs.

I have heard of smokers not wanting to quit since they think they will gain weight.

So, what do we do when we find out we are a substance addict?

Well, it is a sobering moment…a time to re-think a lot of things.

If someone never smokes a cigarette, they will never crave nicotine.

For someone who was addicted at some point in the past, if they take even one puff of that cigarette, they could revert to the addiction. That is how powerful the addiction is.

So why do people like to smoke in the first place?

There are "good" things that come from smoking such as it being relaxing and calming.

In fact, there were many times when I worked at the government office that I wished I was a smoker.

They were allowed to take 10 min "smoke breaks" every hour, and I could have used a break too!

They always seemed relaxed, just standing, or sitting having their break while I had to keep working in my cubicle.

Interestingly, when I started to see my carb addiction in this light, maybe I was having my own kind of "smoke break" but instead I was nibbling on my muffin, or sipping on my sweetened tea, latte or can of pop…my "snack break".

I guess I was a carb addict, and I WAS getting a break!

So, can we equate carb addiction to these other substances in terms of quitting?

Can we try to quit eating and drinking all the carbs we have been used to...all the muffins, chips, fries, and beers?

Can even one bite, snack, or meal with sugar, high carb, or processed foods make us also revert to our carb addiction?

I needed to learn more.

We would never tell a smoker to just will themselves to not smoke again (or tell an alcoholic to stop drinking).

Society now knows how addictive nicotine (and alcohol) can be. Yet 50-70 years ago, the addictive nature of smoking was not so well known.

In fact, doctors would recommend smoking for people who wanted to lose weight or keep the weight off!

It seems utterly ridiculous nowadays to think of that.

Now, once I started to see how addictive sugar was, it made all of this so much clearer.

All these substance addictions have something in common. They mess with our brains and bodies and are VERY hard to quit.

As I look back on it, it was sometime in March of 2021 when the turning point came for me.

I wanted this to be my LAST diet – the last time I lost this weight!

My new goal was to become a "recovered carb addict" and to become "carb sober" as much as possible.

For me, once I saw it like I was becoming a recovering smoker or a recovering alcoholic, I knew that this diet and way of eating was different from all the others I had tried.

Hearing that it takes smokers 4 - 7 times before they are successful at quitting smoking made me think of all the times I had been on those yo-yo diets.

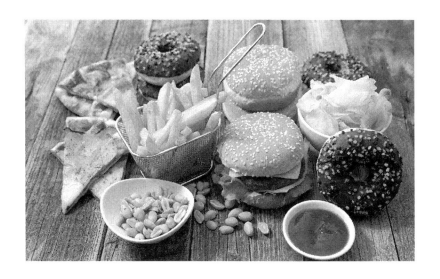

How do I overcome my carb addiction?

RECOMMENDED

"Addiction explained by the Carb Addiction Doc - Dr. Rob Cywes" from the **Carnivore Yogi** YouTube channel.[43]

The main root of my carb addiction was not my fault...the desserts, cereals, breads, and fruit were fed to me before I was at an age to decide. I just kept up the eating habits throughout my life without questioning them.

But now that I knew I had a carb addiction, it was my responsibility to address it if I wanted to be healthier as I got older.

Looking back, it has been an amazing journey to start to learn and experience this breakthrough!

It has been so liberating, and yet I know I must stay vigilant.

It's the sugar that makes the body crave more...not my lack of willpower or lack of self-discipline!

Keep the sugar away to keep the carb cravings at bay.

Keeping the sugar/high carb/processed foods out of sight, out of the cupboards, out of the fridge and freezer and off the grocery list has made a huge difference.

When someone quits smoking, they throw away all the packs of cigarettes.

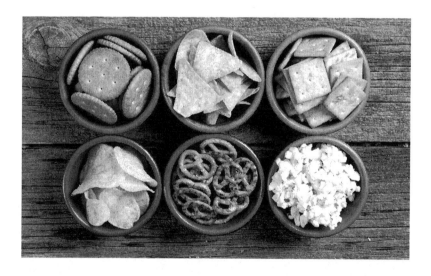

When someone quits carbs, tossing out all the bread, pasta, crackers, cookies, candy and cereals that once filled our cupboards helps so much in curbing the carb addiction.

It will feel like an uphill battle to try to quit just through sheer willpower.

We are not tempted to overeat on healthy carbs such as vegetables. It is the overly sweet carbs and processed carbs that we can't stop eating.

A smoker throws "money" away when they toss out their last packs of cigarettes.

So too, I threw some "money" in the garbage when I threw out much of the processed foods I had bought (I also I donated some of it to another family).

That money was only thrown away once though, since I changed what foods I started to buy in the first place.

Think about it - all the food in our fridge, freezer and cupboards is food we chose to buy.

We chose to put it in the shopping cart, pay for it and bring it home.

So, from now on, we can make better choices at the grocery store and eliminate the temptation, at the source!

RECOMMENDED

"Ep:130 What You Must Know About Yourself Before You Start Keto Or Recover From A Relapse - R Cywes" from the **Dr. Cywes the #CarbAddictionDoc** YouTube channel. [44]

When I heard about how the average overweight person snacks up to 12 times a day, which is similar to someone smoking 12 times a day, it made me stop and think.

Every time food enters my mouth, I should see that as a meal, not just a snack that somehow does not count.

Every time I take a sip of my "double-double" coffee, or pop, or beer, my body sees this as having a small meal and stimulates an insulin response.

Was I giving my insulin a rollercoaster ride all throughout the day? YES!

The taste, the flavour, the smell was a hit to my brain…what a rush!

Also, when I look back, I was using carbs as a mechanism for relaxation instead of eating foods to fuel my body properly.

Not caring about my body's needs was a mistake that was going to be making life even more difficult as I got older.

Whatever I overate, that was my addiction and for me, it always involved carbs.

I imagined the smaller body I would have once I lost the weight and I started to turn a corner and change my relationship with food.

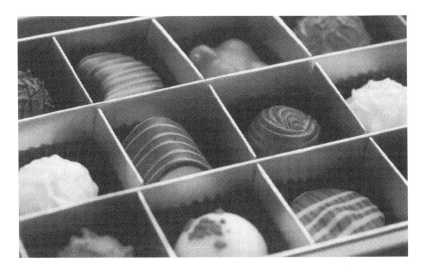

WHAT IS MY RELATIONSHIP WITH FOOD?

Every person has different addictions within the carb categories. I asked myself…what is my specific relationship with each food?

Starting to categorize foods as "risky" instead of "cheat" foods, became a helpful guide. I made a list of foods that were the most addictive to me…that I craved and couldn't stop eating once I started.

The high-risk foods were high in carbs and could be seen as smoking when I used that comparison.

The medium risk foods I could compare to e-cigarettes, nicotine gum, or non-alcoholic beer, for those with smoking or alcoholic addictions.

The low-risk foods were like basically not smoking at all since they didn't make me want to overeat them.

I'm sure all carb-addicts will have their own favourites.

For me, this was my list.

LOW RISK CARBS
(no chance of overeating)

* Potatoes
* Sweet potatoes
* Vegetables

MEDIUM RISK CARBS

(some chance of overeating)

I can graze and snack on it before I know the limit and then eat too much…

- Dairy (pudding, flavoured yogurt)
- Tortillas
- Rice and pasta
- Fruit
- Juices/smoothies

VERY RISKY CARBS

(high chance of overeating)

I find it hard to stop eating or only have 1 bite:

- Desserts
- Breads
- Candy
- Chocolate

In the early days of trying to eat low carb, unless my daughter was standing next to me and watched me only have 1 bite, I literally had to stop eating those VERY RISKY foods.

Just like a former smoker would not trust themselves to just have one drag on a cigarette…it was just too risky.

Now, having come this far, I don't want to undo all the hard effort I put into kicking this carb addiction. Starting over would be so discouraging for me.

Thinking back to 15 years ago, after we had come back from Brazil, we had cable TV for while. I remember watching a British TV show called *"You Are What You Eat"* with Gillian McKeith. [18]

At the beginning of each show, she would talk to her guests about what they had eaten in the previous week.

Gillian would even go to their homes and look in their fridges and cupboards. They could not hide what they ate!

Then the next week they would come back to her, and she would have somehow rounded up a sample of all the foods they had eaten in the previous week.

I will never forget looking at the table full of food…and almost all of it was CARBS!

Even though I don't endorse everything Gillian talks about, I recommend you check out her show on YouTube. Just seeing that table full of food is enough to get the picture.

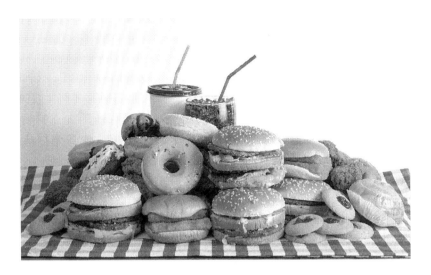

I have thought of that show many times over the past decade and there are times when I picture someone doing that for me…laying out all the food I ate in the previous 7 days.

I would feel shame at how unbalanced it was…way too many carbs in comparison to healthy protein, healthy fat, and vegetables that would be better for me to eat.

For instance, if I put all the brownies I have consumed over the years on a table…well, it would probably overflow and fill up a whole room!

This visual picture has been helpful to make me see that in my 50+ years on this earth, I have had enough brownies for one lifetime!

The same goes for bread, donuts, cookies, cakes and candy!

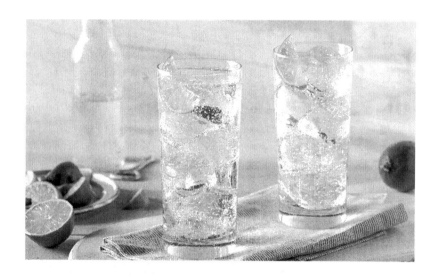

WHAT IS A LOW-CARB FLU?

Not surprisingly, for those of us who have a carb addiction
(not everyone does), I have found that it's getting rid of the
high carb foods that is the only way to really "quit."

When people with other substance addictions try to quit, there
are drawbacks.

If they quit "cold turkey", they can be miserable for several
days or even weeks.

This is also true for sugar and carbs. If we stop eating them
too quickly, we will have flu-like symptoms which can be
very unpleasant.

I have experienced this many times over the years when I would start a diet. I would feel terrible for a couple days. It literally felt like I had the flu.

Since I started listening to Dr. Jason Fung, Dr. Robert Cywes and Dr. Berry and others, I knew this might happen too, so I tried to come off of carbs more slowly.

Some of them recommend changing one thing each week.

For example, back in 2012, I switched from coke to diet coke when I went Paleo. Then I stopped drinking pop all together.

After that, my drink of choice had been juice and smoothies. I would thaw frozen fruit and mix it in a blender with fruit juice. I saw it as a "healthy" drink.

But it was loaded with way too many carbs, especially since I would sip on it, making my insulin rise and fall.

So, I slowly switched to other flavoured drinks, carbonated water and eventually off the carbonated drinks altogether.

Over several weeks, I slowly implemented small habits to begin to replace those drinks.

I knew I would not be drinking these on a long term basis, but it really helped in the first few weeks and months.

I tried to have between 6-8 different types and flavours available.

These are some examples:

- Sparkling water
- Mineral water
- Club soda
- Artificial flavouring to mix with water

Remember…this is only a TEMPORARY thing since artificial sweeteners are not recommended to consume on a regular basis, especially not for children and teens.

Weaning off these artificial sweetened and carbonated drinks took me several months.

Now, regarding foods, I started to give up morning toast with jam or honey and just had toast with butter.

I would alternate with cereal or flavoured yogurt. Then after a few weeks I started having eggs and bacon without the toast.

Then eventually I didn't even eat breakfast once I chose to follow the intermittent fasting option.

The goal of all of this was long term freedom from carb addiction. Being able to come off the addiction slowly was important for me so that I would not get that low carb flu.

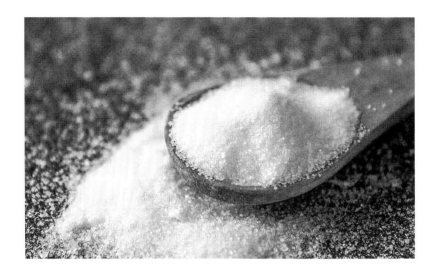

WHAT ABOUT SALT?

Because the SAD diet includes so much processed and refined foods, there is enough salt in that diet.

But once we start cooking from scratch and use one-ingredient foods, we will need to add more salt to our diet.

We can get headaches and lose electrolytes if we don't add more salt.

It is recommended to have pickle juice, bone broth, electrolyte drops or even some grains of salt added to water in order to get enough salt during the day.

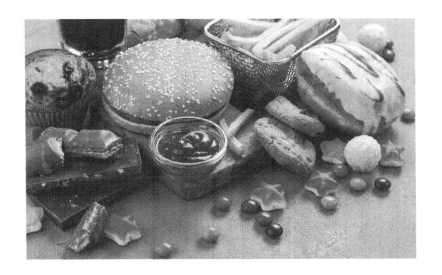

10 - SNACKS

HOW DO YOU OVERCOME EMOTIONAL EATING?

Replacing high carb foods with other emotional regulation techniques helped fill the void...I call them my "carb patches" (like nicotine patches for people who are quitting smoking).

As I learned more, I became very aware that I had usually used carbs as a way to relax.

The truth of the matter is when I started to get the picture that no diet will be successful for me unless I faced the fact that I had an addiction, then I started to see it in a new light.

This helped me admit I needed to grieve…saying goodbye to the foods that once gave me comfort.

I needed to remove the carbs and replace them with things that did not hurt my body.

This quote has stuck with me:

"Snacking is always an emotional event."

Dr. Robert Cywes

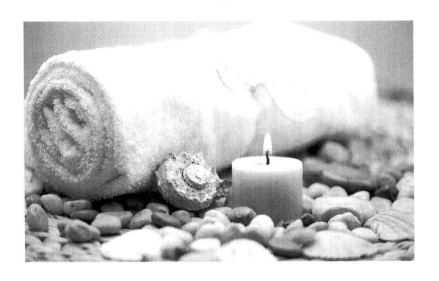

WHAT IS A "BRIDGE" IN TERMS OF CARB ADDICTION?

When I first heard the YouTube video by Dr. Cywes where he talked about the "bridge", it made so much sense!

RECOMMENDED

"EP:04 snacks vs bridges" from the **Dr. Cywes the #CarbAddictionDoc** YouTube channel. [40]

As I mentioned in the section about the low carb flu, having some 0-carb drinks in the fridge to "snack" on when I felt like a treat was so helpful at the beginning

These were "bridges" and were something to help me as I kicked the carb-addiction habits. Put simply, there are healthy ways to get an endorphin hit instead of through carb-heavy beverages and foods.

I found things to replace the carb-endorphin rush that used to have a big place in my life. I found a "bridge" to get me over the hump till I needed "another hit."

Dr. Cywes recommends making rituals or routines…sipping black coffee or unsweetened tea, sipping on some type of liquid that has 0 carbs. Replace, don't deprive. He talks about a "mind cleansing moment," like a smoker's break.

RECOMMENDED

Ketogenic Rules for: Drinking and Hydration" from the **Dr. Cywes the #CarbAddictionDoc** YouTube channel.[41]

These are 5 things that could count as an "action snack":

* Creative arts and crafts
* Exercise and fitness
* Meditation
* Connecting with people
* Healthy pleasure and passion

Here is a list of 25 non-food related ways we can find emotional regulations to "snack" on in order to have a "mental health fix":

1. Listen to music
2. Connect with friends
3. Avoid stress
4. Brush teeth
5. Write in a journal
6. Drink tea
7. Get a massage
8. Stretch
9. Garden
10. Take a shower or bath
11. Do yoga
12. Go out with friends
13. Enjoy family time
14. Watch a movie
15. Do some Pilates
16. Learn a new hobby
17. Take a nap
18. Listen to comedy
19. Play with a pet
20. Get out in the sunshine
21. Drink water
22. Practice a musical instrument
23. Watch a movie
24. Take a walk
25. Chew gum

Of course, there are numerous other things that could be added to this list.

Getting rid of things that will set us back is helpful – things that remind us of the most tempting carbs.

I really struggled with this at the beginning.

Many mornings I would feel like giving up and having breakfast even if I was not hungry. Or I would snack and overeat on nuts and then have a terrible stomach ache.

Other times, I would justify baking a Keto snack, telling myself it was allowed since it was not made with wheat flour. Then, after I had consumed way too much, I would blame myself and feel shame.

These times came and went, when I had willpower and when I gave in to my old habits.

Picking myself up, choosing to make better choices, I slowly changed my habits.

And it got easier.

We can all expect setbacks when we change habits in our live. But it gives us an opportunity to try again, and again.

Some people find journaling helps. I found keeping busy and occupied with fun activities or work projects really helped me.

The other people in our household might not be on the same weight loss and health journey that we are on.

I was lucky in that while I was losing the weight, I only had my youngest daughter living with me.

Because of our small household, I was not as tempted as I would have been in the past if there were a lot more people in the house.

As we change, the people in our life will change in response to how we act. Others will learn from our behaviours and see the great results we are having.

Though it can be stressful on our relationships to change old habits and behaviours, if we are doing them for the right reasons, then they benefit everyone around us too.

I know my children were very grateful to see me so motivated towards my goal of getting healthier.

Some relationships can help us make this big lifestyle change. Maybe finding a weight loss buddy that we can check in with regularly could really help.

Of course, the best way to stay motivated is to keep remembering our "WHY" for weight loss. Why do we want to lose the weight and take back control of our eating?

When I do an internet search for diabetes, fatty liver disease, insulin resistance, inflammation, cancer, etc., it helps remind me why I am quitting carbs and not wanting to be obese anymore.

I am happy with baby steps that walk me away from health problems and towards longevity.

Is it worth kicking the carb addiction? YES!!!!

The reward is getting to the place where I no longer obsess about what to eat or when to eat. I don't crave the carbs anymore!

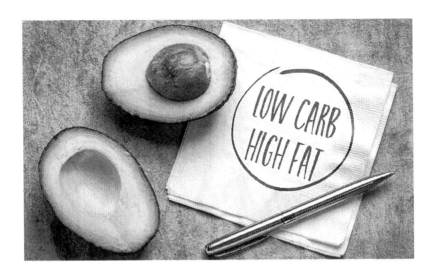

11 - LOW CARB HIGH FAT

WHAT IS A LCHF DIET?

NOTE: Please make sure you first read my disclaimers at the start of this book before you start any diet.

There are many diets that fall under the category of low carb, high fat (LCHF). Diets such as Atkins, Paleo, Keto and AIP for example. The diet I started in 2021 was a combination of Keto and AIP.

The Keto diet is a way of eating that helps take away the hunger and cravings. Generally, under 50 grams of carbs per day counts as being in ketosis. [26]

By eating low carb, those nasty carb cravings are gone. It truly is amazing once you experience it.

DEFINITIONS

"A ketogenic diet – or keto diet – is a low-carb, high-fat diet. It can be effective for weight loss and certain health conditions, something that's been demonstrated in many studies. A keto diet is especially useful for losing excess body fat without hunger, and for improving type 2 diabetes or metabolic syndrome. On a keto diet, you cut way back on carbohydrates, also known as carbs, in order to burn fat for fuel." [7]

You know that feeling when you can't stop thinking about a certain snack in the fridge or ingredient on the shelf, or a restaurant you want to go to?

That was how I was, all day long!

But, once I started eating Keto and low carb, I started thinking about food less. I will never forget realizing one day that I literally would forget to eat – it was a totally new reality for me.

After I stopped eating breakfasts, the day would fly by, and I had not even gone in the kitchen!

It was liberating…not being tied to the food, being able to stop nibbling and grazing.

My body got used to eating fewer carbs and so I craved carbs less and less. Discovering what foods made me hungry helped show me which foods had more carbs.

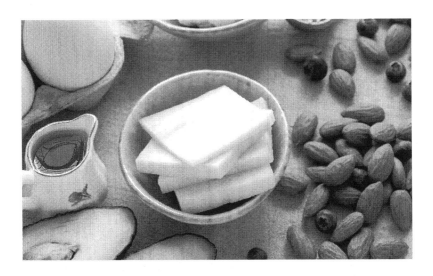

WHAT ABOUT FATS AND OILS?

RECOMMENDED

"LCUSA - WPB 2019 - final session" from the **LowCarbUSA** YouTube channel. [39]

When I ate foods that had a higher fat content, the less I would feel hunger.

Here is a list of healthy fats:

* Full-fat dairy
* Butter and ghee
* Coconut oil
* Olive oil
* Nuts and seeds

These are all fats that I learned are healthier than the artificial and highly processed foods that most diets recommend.

When I look at the ingredients on margarine, most of it is not natural…but instead chemicals to make it taste like the real thing. Why not just eat the real thing?

The foods that had low or no carbs and higher fat contents, I would not be tempted to overeat.

For instance, whenever I ate a steak, I would feel full, and I just wasn't tempted to overeat.

I learned that if I didn't crave the food, it was a good indication that there were few or no carbs and more healthy fats, and enough nutrition for my body to stay healthy.

My body had its own built-in way of telling me not to overeat them. And, as I started eating lower carb foods every day, I actually reset my pallet.

The key was being aware of how every different food affected my body.

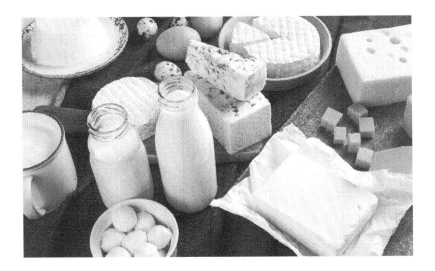

Let's say each time we drink a glass of milk, we get a stomach-ache. This is a sign worth listening to, and many people who have a dairy intolerance know they have to consume less dairy or completely eliminate dairy foods altogether.

For other people, dairy is fine, and it does not cause physical symptoms when they drink milk or eat cheese.

This is one way they listen to their bodies.

In a similar way, when we start to be aware of the cravings for high-carb, low fat foods, the LCHF way of eating will make it so much easier since there will be fewer carbs in our diet.

Pretty soon, we won't like the cravings.

The carb cravings will distract us from work or life.

The cravings will make us think about food and want to go make or buy the food we are craving.

Then, it is a slippery slope back to being a carb addict again.

It has been so helpful for me to re-educate myself having grown up with the typical western food pyramid where carbs were the most important thing.

RECOMMENDED

"Ketogenic Rules For: A Healthy Liver" from the **Dr. Cywes the #CarbAddictionDoc** YouTube channel. [42]

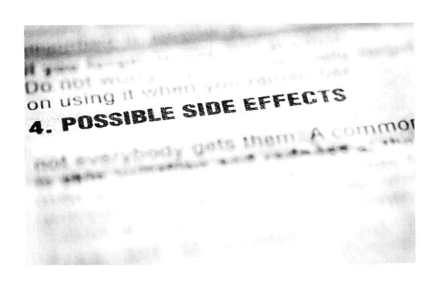

4. POSSIBLE SIDE EFFECTS

WHAT ARE SOME SIDE EFFECTS OF LCHF?

When I started eating low carb and doing intermitted fasting every day, after about 3 months I had significant hair loss. This lasted for almost 4 months.

In hindsight, I should have started taking biotin pills and collagen powder every day, but I didn't until my hair was noticeably thinner.

Thankfully, the very first week I started with the biotin pills and collagen powder, I could see hair regrowth and now it is fuller and has all grown back.

Another side effect when I started eating low carb was having itchy skin. It was only on the parts of my body where I had the most stored fat.

I would wake up in the night feeling very itchy. Reading other people's experiences in the Facebook groups, I knew this was part of the process and to not worry about it.

Applying moisturizing cream helped a lot. And after a few weeks, the itching disappeared.

Other people have different side effects from losing weight or going low carb. Finding resources online and groups where people share their stories is very helpful to get through these times and know we are not alone in our struggle.

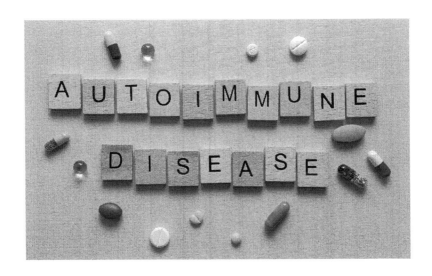

12 - AIP AND GUT HEALTH

WHAT IS THE AIP DIET?

Proceed with caution!
The AIP diet is an elimination diet and being on
it for too long can lead to malnutrition. It is not
intended to be a long-term diet.

Ok, now that we have started with caution, here is a definition
of the Autoimmune Protocol Diet (AIP).

DEFINITIONS

"Autoimmune Protocol Diet (AIP): It's based on the idea that certain foods inflame your gut, and that eliminating them may ease autoimmune symptoms. Once you've stopped eating and drinking all of these things, you wait to see if your autoimmune symptoms improve. If they do, you slowly start to eat the nixed foods again, one at a time, to find out if any of them trigger your symptoms. The idea is that you'll learn which foods to stay away from. This type of eating plan is called an elimination diet. People usually stay on an elimination diet for only about 4 to 8 weeks." [27]

While primarily following the Keto diet to lose the weight, I also combined it with the Autoimmune Protocol diet (AIP).

This diet is similar in that it is low carb, but they only recommend being on it for a few weeks or months at a time since it is even more restrictive than Keto.

Basically, the AIP diet eliminates all foods that are known to cause inflammation for some people and it is recommended for those who want to "heal their gut."

This means temporarily eliminating foods such as dairy, nuts, grains, sugars, eggs, alcohol, chocolate, processed foods, junk food, and pop.

Some people will go even further and eliminate foods such as potatoes, peppers, and tomatoes.

While eating AIP, I primarily eat only cooked vegetable, meat, bone broth, and a small amount of fruit – all of these are easy to digest.

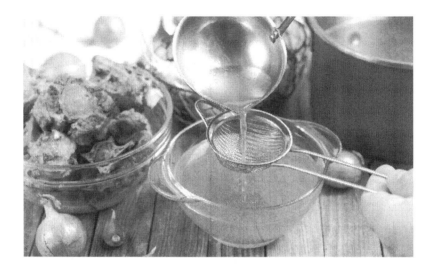

You can probably see why this restrictive diet is not recommended for very long.

It's very boring (so not sustainable or practical) and lacks certain essential vitamins and minerals…but it certainly does heal the gut, and help our bodies recover from eating foods that may be causing bad reactions.

RECOMMENDED

"Leaky Gut Got You Down? How to Reverse Autoimmune Disease" from the **CBN News** YouTube channel. [4]

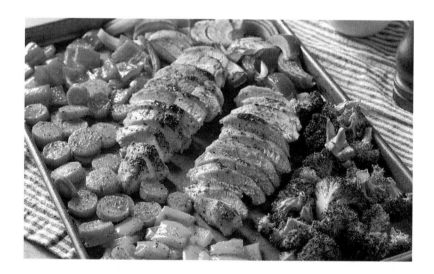

WHY GO ON THE AIP DIET?

In Chapter 5, I talked about having a mini stroke. Before my stroke, I had heart palpitations and arrhythmia for several years. After my stroke, I kept having these issues.

During the months that followed, I went off the Paleo diet and started getting more tests including going to see a cardiologist.

After a stress test, adrenaline test, and blood work all came back with normal results, the cardiologist said that it must just be early menopause symptoms. However, up till that point I had no other signs that I was perimenopausal.

So why was I having these heart palpitations? I started doing my own research.

I came across an article that talked about caffeine and food additives that were in soy sauce and other chemicals, and that these could be causing some people to have heart palpitations and arrhythmia.

A few summers earlier, I remembered when my son, who was 18 years old at the time, had gone on the AIP diet for 8 weeks. He had been having terrible stomach aches and also dealt with acne.

We all saw such a big change in him after he tried the AIP diet. After just 2 months, he completely cured his acne and stomach aches.

After doing more of my own research on elimination diets including the GAPS diet [6] and AIP diets, I decided I would give it a try.

I prepped for a few weeks in anticipation of the diet, knowing it was very restrictive.

After just 3 weeks on AIP, my heart palpitations were almost completely gone. It was unbelievable!

It felt like I had reset my system and healed my gut. I was not waking up with my heart pounding.

So, in 2021, remembering how this had helped me in the past, I decided to combine the Keto and AIP diets to help me lose weight.

I lessened the amount of nuts and dairy I was consuming but increased the amount of fruit and potatoes.

My goal was to not become malnourished as I had on the Paleo diet. So, I tried to eat a large variety of meats and vegetables. Variety was the key (and continues to be as I maintain my weight loss).

After I reached my goal weight, I brought back some more nuts and high-fat dairy and kept the home-prepared potatoes and sweet potatoes as well.

By alternating meals and mixing it up, it helped to keep my body guessing and not overloading it with just a few types of food or cause it to become malnourished again.

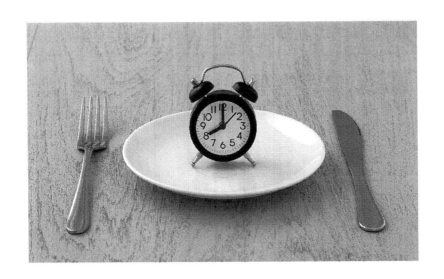

13 - INTERMITTENT FASTING

WHAT IS INTERMITTENT FASTING?

RECOMMENDED

"Beginning Fasting (What to Expect) | Jason Fung" from the **Jason Fung** YouTube channel. [12]

Historically, humans have endured times of feasting and famine. When there is a lot of food available, we can store the extra energy as fat which can be used up later during times of scarcity.

Stored fat is actually amazing! It is good to have some extra fat on our bodies, but too much fat is harmful.

DEFINITIONS

"Intermittent fasting simply allows the body to use its stored sources of energy – blood sugar and body fat. This is an entirely normal process and humans have evolved these storage forms of food energy precisely so that we can fast for hours or days without detrimental health consequences. Blood sugar and body fat is merely stored food energy to fuel the body when food is not readily available. By fasting, we are lowering blood sugar and body fat by using them precisely for the reason we store them." [32]

Intermittent fasting is choosing to only eat during specific times of the day.

RECOMMENDED

"The Physiology of Intermittent Fasting (Science) | Jason Fung" from the **Jason Fung** YouTube channel. [10]

We can have a time of fasting and then an "eating window". This refers to how much time we allow ourselves to eat, in between our fasting time.

Just like normal eating schedules for breakfast at a certain time or lunch at noon, etc., now we can learn to schedule in our fasting times.

At the beginning, it was helpful to delay my meals.

If I normally ate lunch at noon, then waiting till one o'clock wasn't too hard. I would do that for a few days and then push it to two o'clock. That is when I would have my first meal.

Then I would fast until 6 pm and then have my second meal.

This meant I was restricting my eating to two times within 24 hours. I also did not snack in between those two meals.

RECOMMENDED

"Intermittent Fasting: Fad or Future? | Jason Fung"
from the **Jason Fung** YouTube channel. [11]

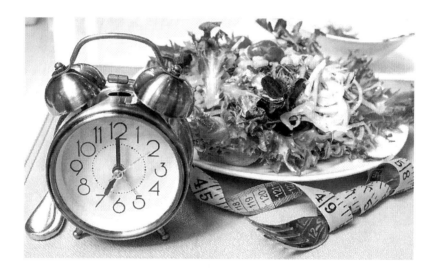

WHAT IS EXTENDED FASTING?

When you don't eat for more than 24 hours, it is called extended fasting.

As I mentioned in Chapter 2, I tried it once in high school as a way to lose weight by only drinking water for 5 days.

I will never forget how it impacted me, not just in losing weight but in how I felt.

The first day was normal. The second and third days I had the low carb flu (see Chapter 9) and I felt very weak. But, by the fourth and fifth days, I remember how much energy I had.

RECOMMENDED

"Dr Jason Fung [Benefits Of Longer Fasts]" from the **Weight Loss Motivation** YouTube channel. [15]

In the past year, I tried extended fasting three separate times.

It was near the beginning of when I was eating low carb and so I was not totally used to the Keto diet.

I made it to 36 hrs., 40 hrs., and 44 hrs. with only water. I left about 3 weeks between each of these attempts at extended fasting. However, each time I had headaches, and had the low-carb flu and felt weak.

At the start, I did not understand much about electrolytes and how we need to add more salt when we take away processed foods from our diets.

After those attempts at extended fasting, I only did intermittent fasting up till 23 hours, or one-meal-a-day (OMAD).

I was still able to lose the weight without any further extended fasts.

In general, its recommended to mix up OMAD and two-meals-a-day (2MAD), but extended fasts can be included as well.

Here is an example of an extended fasting schedule. I have not tried these, but many people in the Facebook communities talk about how successful these can be:

SCHEDULE 30/16/30/16

- Fasting 30 hours = Monday lunch to Tuesday Supper

- Fasting 16 hours = Tuesday supper to Wednesday lunch

- Fasting 30 hours = Wednesday lunch to Thursday supper

- Fasting 16 hours = Thursday supper to Friday lunch

- Then on the weekend, there can be two days of 2MAD

RECOMMENDED

"When Should We Eat On A Keto Diet? Mindblow Time - by Robert Cywes" from the **Dr. Cywes the #CarbAddictionDoc** YouTube channel. [45]

I will say here that when I tried extended fasting, I saw how it could make me want to binge eat and since that eating disorder is in my history, I wanted to avoid that temptation to slip back into old patterns.

I may try it in the future again to help with autophagy[34] but for now, I am fine with 2MAD and OMAD.

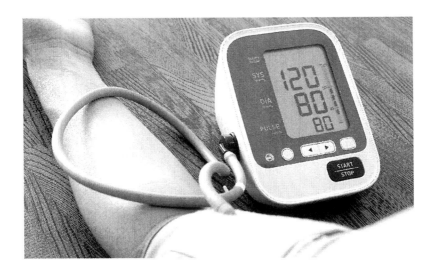

How will intermittent fasting improve my health?

RECOMMENDED

"Intermittent Fasting Dr Jason Fung [5 Stages of Fasting]" from the **Weight Loss Motivation** YouTube channel. [14]

Even though I primarily talk about finding weight loss success, some people find out about LCHF diets and intermittent fasting even though they are already at their goal weight (and maybe have not had a carb addiction to deal with).

As I learned more, I was surprised by what can happen in our bodies when we give our digestion a rest and don't graze on food all day long.

There can be very positive results achieved from intermittent fasting according to the Fasting Method blog as outlined below:

DEFINITIONS

"The Science of Intermittent Fasting" [32]:
* *Lowered blood insulin and glucose levels*
* *Reduced hemoglobin*
* *Reduced medication dependency*
* *Improved blood pressure (hypertension)*
* *Improved cholesterol levels*
* *Improved mental clarity and concentration*
* *Increased energy*
* *Increased growth hormone*
* *Increased longevity*
* *Activated cellular cleansing by stimulating autophagy*
* *Reduction of inflammation*

DEFINITIONS

"Autophagy is the natural cellular recycling process that rids our body of old or malfunctional protein. This sets in motion the process of rejuvenation as our body rebuilds new proteins to replace the old ones. Autophagy is a powerful method of healing and is best activated by fasting." [34]

After barely touching the surface of the benefits of intermittent fasting, I will just encourage you to review the recommended links and resources since the experts are the one with all the knowledge in these areas.

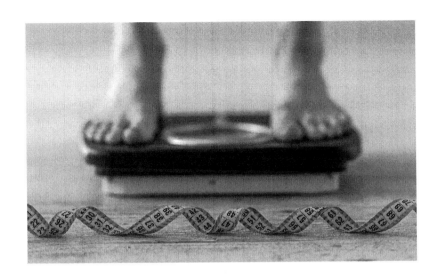

14 - WEIGH SCALES AND CALORIES

WHAT IS BMI?

DEFINITIONS

"Body mass index (BMI) uses weight and height to estimate body fat. A high BMI is associated with an increased risk for chronic diseases such as heart disease, high blood pressure, and type 2 diabetes in adults. BMI provides a reasonable estimate of body fat for most people." [21]

The BMI ratings are as follows:

- Normal weight = 18-24
- Overweight = 25-29
- Obese = over 30

I am 5 feet, 5 inches tall (165 cm). At various times in my life I have had a BMI of 18 or 19 but never stayed there for very long. When I was at my heaviest, (210 lbs) my BMI was over 35.

Now that I have reached my goal weight and am a bit lower even (126 lbs) my BMI is 21. It is good to see that I am within the normal BMI for my height and age.

RECOMMENDED

"Fasting Vs. Cutting Calories? (The scientific advantage) | *Jason Fung"* from the **Jason Fung** YouTube channel. [9]

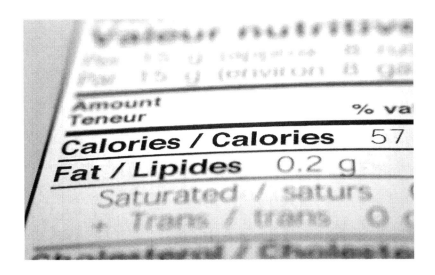

WHEN DO I HAVE TO COUNT CALORIES?

Do you ever dream of losing weight without needing to count calories?

Counting calories is tedious! I have done it so many times over the years.

But this time around, I only needed to count calories at the beginning and then only to estimate how fast I wanted to lose the weight.

For some reference, this helped me at the beginning…

There are 3,500 calories per 1 lb of fat.

Our bodies use approx. 1,800 calories just to exist since our brain and organs need calories to function each day.

So, if we don't eat for a whole day (and we would normally eat 1,800 calories), then we will lose around 1/2 lb of fat per day of stored fat (3,500 - 1,800 = 1,800)

If we do an extended fast for 7-days and lose 10 lbs, we have only lost 3 ½ lbs of stored fat. The rest is water and fluid loss but not actual fat from our stored fat cells.

Basically, that is all we have to know about counting calories and we never have to count the calories in food again!

That is one of the best things about this diet/lifestyle.

Now, at the start, I did need to count carbs, but I got the hang of it and eventually, I was only eating foods that didn't have nutritional labels.

Think about that…not needing to look at labels!

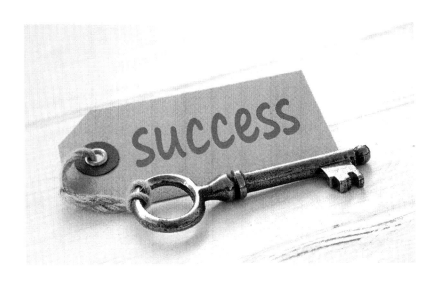

HOW LONG WILL IT TAKE TO LOSE WEIGHT?

When I remembered how many years/decades it took to gain my weight, I knew it would take time for my body to adjust its cells as I started to lose the weight.

Once I stopped the steady supply of carbs/sugar, I started to use up my stored energy (stored fat).

So, when I had my last 45 lbs to lose, I remember trying to reverse engineer how long it would take to reach my goal weight.

I estimated this by calculating how many actual calories of stored fat I needed to NOT eat.

If we normally would eat 1,800 calories daily, then only eating OMAD at 900 calories, we would burn an additional 900 calories of stored fat (1/4 lb).

In 7 days, we would have burned up 6,300 calories which is 1.8 lbs of fat.

Now, when I had 45 lbs left to lose, I calculated it like this.

45 lbs times 3,500 calories per lb equals 157,500 calories.

Therefore, in 1 week of OMAD burning up 6,300 calories (1.8 lbs of stored fat), it would take me 25 weeks to lose 45 lbs.

157,500 divided by 6,300 equals 25 weeks.

I assumed there would be ups and downs, so I allowed myself more than the 25 weeks to lose the 45 lbs.

It took approx. 38 weeks instead of 25 weeks…but I was still thrilled since I ultimately DID reach my goal!!

Note…it is not recommended to do OMAD every day since it is hard to eat enough food during that 1-hour eating window.

Our bodies will slow our metabolism down if we don't eat enough each day since it will go into starvation mode.

Slowing our metabolism is one of the risks of intermittent and extended fasting and why we need to take it seriously and learn about it.

It is VERY important to eat a lot when we do eat…filling up our plate with lots of protein and cooked vegetables especially…and, eating until we are full.

As mentioned earlier, I alternated between 2MAD and OMAD to keep up the variety and to keep my metabolism up.

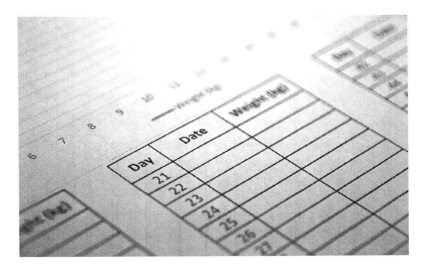

HOW DO I KEEP TRACK OF MY WEIGHT LOSS?

After I had stopped listening to the messaging from the body positivity movement and their aversion to the weigh scale, I purchased a new weigh scale in 2019.

I would weigh myself once in a while, but then in 2021, I started to weigh myself every day.

The best time to weigh myself was in the morning after my shower, but before I had eaten or drank anything. Also, I always weighed myself naked.

This was the easiest ways to have consistency, since food, drink, clothes, and time of day can all add to the number.

Every morning I would enter my weight on the simple chart I had made on my bedroom wall.

This was one of the best things I did...have it on the wall, visible. I would go up and down in weight during the week, but mostly down.

For the first 4 months, I lost some weight every single week.

As I got closer to my goal weight, the weight came off more slowly. Then, I plateaued for a month.

However, I persevered, and would keep weighing myself every morning.

And when I was discouraged, I would simply look back on my chart and see how far I had come.

Daily habits would indeed help me reach my goal…the goal I had set in January of 2021 to lose that last 45 lbs (180 lbs down to 135 lbs)

Amazingly, after I reached the 135 lbs goal weight, I realized that I wanted to keep going.

So many times in the past, I would have celebrated my weight loss and rewarded myself with "cheat meals", gone off the diet and gained the weight back.

This time was different. I decided to keep at it.

I finally weighed in at 130 lbs in November of 2021 and then 128 lbs by December of 2021. I stopped weighing myself every day and only did it once every week or two.

In conclusion, for some of us, the weight scale is a good tool to help keep track of successes in the goal to get to a "normal weight" range.

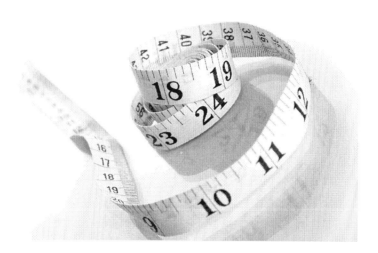

WHAT ARE "NON-SCALE" VICTORIES?

"Non-scale" victories refer to things that don't relate to the weigh scale that we can be grateful for while we are losing weight.

Here are a few examples:

- Changing body measurements
- Fitting into smaller clothes
- Having fewer wrinkles
- Having fewer "ailments"
- Reducing inflammation
- Going off of certain meds
- Improving moods
- Learning to cook from scratch

- Saving money on food
- Thinking less about food
- Learning about my body and nutrition
- Conquering carb addiction habits
- Feeling a sense of accomplishment
- Feeling more confidence
- Feeling excitement in future goals

While I was losing the weight, all the things listed above were victories that I could celebrate.

These were things that showed me that what I was doing was working…intermittent fasting and low-carb eating was the way for me to achieve weight loss success!

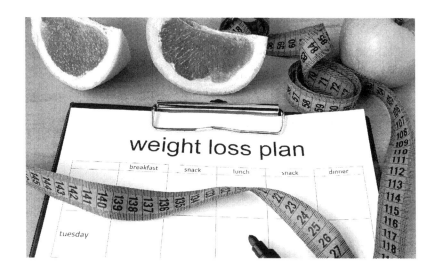

15 - GOALS AND PLANS

WHEN WILL I SEE RESULTS?

If your goal is weight loss and you could lose 1 lb per week, would you be happy with that result? That equals 52 lbs in a year.

Remember, we don't put on all our weight in a short time and so it takes a while to take it off permanently.

I am realizing that the only way to make it permanent is to deal with the root cause of why we have access fat in the first place (which I talk about in previous chapters).

If we have a 3-month, 6-month, or 12-month goal, or even a 2-year goal, then we can plan our weight loss success story AHEAD OF TIME!

It's like working backwards (I do like to reverse engineer things!).

Back in the beginning of 2021, I imagined 8 months down the road. What size did I want to be wearing in 8 months once I had reached my goal weight?

Since it had taken me 4 years to gain the 80 lbs, I couldn't expect to lose those 80 lbs overnight…AND keep them off.

Ultimately, I had to change the behaviours and habits that made me gain the 80 lbs in the first place.

Of course, I needed to change my thinking, my routines, and habits, and increase my knowledge of why I had so much difficulty in stopping my carb addiction.

When thinking about this whole weight loss process, the following list helped with staying on track:

- Remember I was worthy
- Tiny daily steps add up to big results
- Deciding what I really wanted
- I was not too old to reinvent myself

As humans, we have always needed to keep evolving. If we didn't keep evolving and learning, our species would have died out a long time ago.

The ebb and flow of life shows us that when we catch a glimpse of what possibilities exist, we want to evolve into being a better human. It's in our nature.

Our mind controls our behaviour and our behaviour creates our experiences.

We may feel like victims, but we can be courageous people AT THE SAME TIME, not letting "victim-hood" define us.

When we acknowledge that we may have childhood food traumas, eating disorders or were part of that infamous "clean-your-plate" club, we can learn healthy ways to deal with our emotions instead of through carb addiction.

Once we realize we have experienced the harmful effects of decades of that carb addiction, we can take matters into our own hands and change our ways.

In reading what I have experienced and the success I have had, hopefully you can see how I have been able to move forward, move on, think differently and in doing so, change my future.

In the past year, I have accomplished things that, only a couple of years ago, I never thought I could.

Like an iceberg, where only a small portion sits visible above the surface of the ocean, making changes to our thinking involves a whole lot of work, under the surface.

Any of the big changes I've made in my life involved literally hundreds of hours of time dedicated to learning new ways of thinking.

I see a cycle where I have a deep, insatiable desire to learn something new…to change my present and future.

Then, I will spend most of my waking hours researching, reading, listening, watching, and talking about the new idea, skill, dream, passion, drive, or goal.

This is what I did when learning about intermittent fasting, Keto, AIP, etc. I immerse myself in those topics, learning all that my mind could hold.

The learning curve was VERY steep at the beginning. But then I hit the top of the curve and found I could lessen my research and put into practice what I had learned...

And the ride down the other side of the learning curve was great. I saw results!

Now, I am rewarded with clarity and yes, my experiences in life has changed.

And it was worth the time and effort…changing my thinking did, in fact, change my experience.

So, here's to learning something new, to new beginnings, no matter our age.

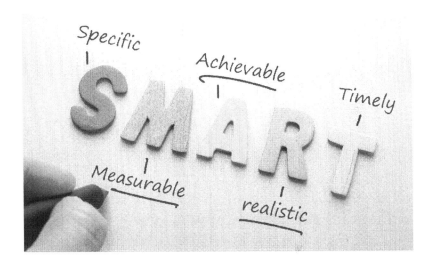

WILL I BE ABLE TO KEEP THE WEIGHT OFF?

This has been a fear of mine…after going on so many diets over the years. I was afraid I would "go off the rails" and gain it all back.

Having S.M.A.R.T. goals helps in everyday life when we are wanting to achieve something.

The same goes for health and weight loss goals.

I feel I have many tools now that I did not have before in order to keep the weight off:

- Online supportive communities in several different Facebook groups
- The success of getting in better health, having a body that I am not embarrassed of
- Having a new smaller wardrobe and keeping my "fat clothes" to remind me how far I've come
- Before, during and after photos to remind me of my achievement
- Not being afraid of small relapses and not giving up if it's not working perfectly
- Aiming to be flexible in my eating habits
- Keeping in mind the I will always have a weakness for carbs (thanks to my 50+ years of carb-eating history)
- Not being afraid of calling myself a "recovering carb addict", just like people who are addicted to nicotine or alcohol also refer to themselves as "in recovery"
- Continuing to learn and stay focused on my goal of being healthy and healing from my carb addiction
- Seeking out like-minded groups, new friends, dates etc. who will not tempt me to fall back into my carb addiction

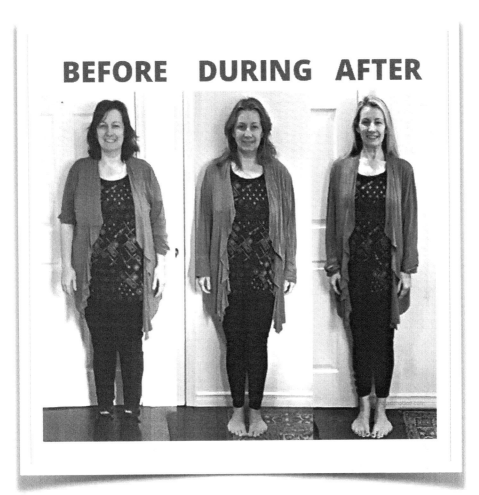

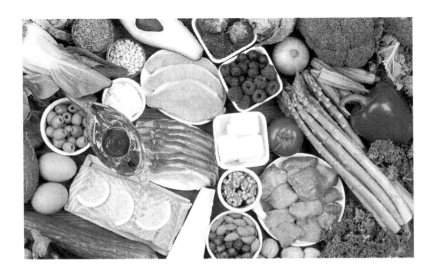

16 - GROCERY LIST

WHAT CAN I EAT ON A LCHF DIET?

Here is a general list of all the foods allowed on the low carb, high fat diet:

- Meats and fish
- Vegetables
- Leafy greens
- Small amounts of berries
- Nuts, seeds including chia seeds
- Eggs
- High-fat dairy and cheese
- Bone broth
- Olive oil, ghee, coconut oil

When I first started eating Keto and eating lower carbs and higher fats, I also started baking with ground almonds, cream cheese, etc. I had learned to bake with ground almonds when I was on the Paleo diet in 2012.

However, since I developed diverticulitis in 2019, my tolerance for Keto baked goods was low.

When I ate them, I would tend to develop diverticulitis flare-ups because I would overeat them. This gave me a stomachache for days.

Even though they did not have the typical white sugar that is in most baking recipes, my brain and body still saw them as sweet snack foods.

Also, when I did try to bake Keto recipes using nut flours and lots of dairy, it stopped me from losing weight. These are not as nutritious as meats and vegetables.

So, I did not eat very many Keto baked goods until I reached my goal weight.

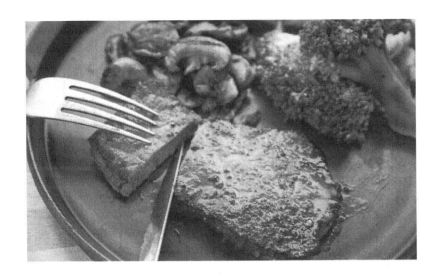

WHAT CAN I EAT ON THE AIP DIET?

Remember, try not to go exclusively AIP for more than a few weeks or months. It is an extreme elimination diet, and you can become malnourished from the lack of variety.

Here are the main categories of foods allowed on the AIP diet:

- Meats and fish
- Vegetables
- Leafy greens
- Fruit (small amounts)
- Bone broth
- Olive oil
- Coconut oil

These are NOT allowed on the AIP diet:

- Eggs
- Dairy
- Nuts
- Seeds
- Grains
- Legumes

As you can see, this is a very restrictive diet.

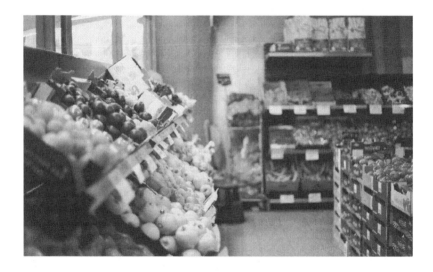

HOW DO I SHOP ON AN LCHF DIET?

Low carb, high fat and Keto diets can be expensive if we live in a place where the meat and fish is pricy.

Grocery shopping is hard when first starting a low carb way of eating, but it gets easier.

When we avoid buying all the snacks, grains, desserts, candy, soft drinks, and beer that we were used to consuming, our grocery bill will be lower.

Also, when we go out to eat at a restaurant, there are fewer options since we have eliminated so many carbs…so we will probably go out to eat less often.

I find it easiest and cheapest to cook from scratch. This will save money in the long run. Being mindful of what we buy at the grocery store is so helpful in keeping us on track and saving money.

When we go to the grocery store, its easy to have a list but then we may end up buying a dozen more things just because they are on sale or look yummy! Good marketing and sales can tempt us into buying more.

Or maybe you can relate to what I used to do.

In the past, since I did not want to waste all the money I had spent:

* If I bought bread, I would eat all the bread
* If I bought chocolate, I would eat all the chocolate
* If I bought desserts, I would eat all the desserts

The food I put in my body started with what I put in my shopping cart!

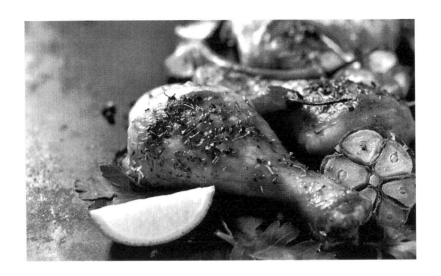

17 - COOKING AND RECIPES

HOW DO YOU COOK LOW-CARB?

Cooking from scratch is the only way to have control over what goes into our bodies.

When we buy pre-made foods, we don't know what has been added, including sugars or highly processed oils and artificial sweeteners.

When we eat at a restaurant, we don't know what quality of ingredients they have used and what chemicals they have added.

Buying whole foods (literally foods that are only one ingredient), we know exactly what we are using to make our recipes.

Have you ever looked at the ingredients list on processed and packaged foods? You can't even read some of the words... they are so long!

And yet it's so easy to just put it in our mouth and eat it since it tastes so good! And 10 min later, we have consumed a whole bag or package.

Food companies hire chemists to make ingredients specifically to be addictive to us so we won't stop eating them and will crave more and buy more.

For myself, I found that learning to cook from scratch was a challenge. I mean, I had learned to cook at cook's training in college and cooked for 3 decades for my family.

But I had not cooked with the goal of "constrained variety" - basically eating as much variety as possible but within the constraints of the LCHF way of eating.

I used to think of dinner needing to include a protein, vegetable, starch (carb), and dessert (carb).

Now, I was doing away with most of the carbs and so had to learn how to cook meals that did not feel monotonous.

Eliminating whole "food groups" with their colour, texture and flavour, I needed to become creative with a smaller list of ingredients.

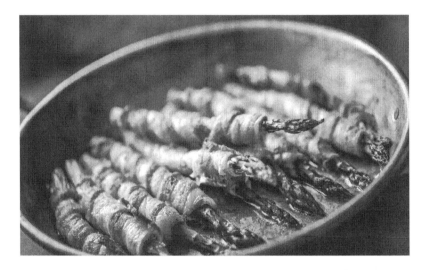

HOW DO YOU COOK FROM SCRATCH?

The LCHF diet is the easiest one to follow along with the addition of a bit of starchy root vegetable and some fruit. I usually bulk-cook and I'm in the kitchen for about 1.5 hours every other day. This saves on time in the kitchen and clean-up.

Typically, this is what a bulk-cooking day looks like for me:

1. Cook 2-3 types of meat. Examples:
   - ✓ slow-cooked pot roast
   - ✓ stir fry beef
   - ✓ roast whole chicken
   - ✓ pan-fried chicken
   - ✓ roast chicken legs
   - ✓ pan-fried salmon or other fish
   - ✓ fried sausage
   - ✓ cooked bacon
2. Roast or steam 2-6 types of vegetables
3. Roast or boil potatoes or sweet potatoes
4. Cut up and wash a head of lettuce or romaine lettuce and store it in salad spinner in the fridge
5. Boil ½ dozen eggs
6. Grate cheese to put on salads, vegetables, or eggs

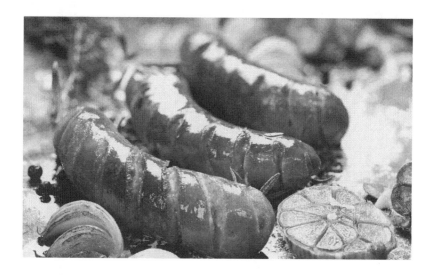

Having this bulk-cooking day allows me to eat for 2-4 days by re-heating.

Of course, some things I am still eating 4-5 days later and other things I need to cook every few days, so there is overlap.

The salads I make each day using the pre-cut lettuce. Then I just need to add raw veggies like cucumbers, tomatoes, peppers, olives, shredded cheese, cut up pickles or sliced boiled eggs.

I try to have a large variety of cooked vegetables over the course of the month, and I rarely eat frozen vegetables as I prefer the raw or roasted flavours.

I do love gravy and cheese sauce, so I do allow myself a small amount of flour or cornstarch (carbs) to help thicken these.

The amount of flour I consume in these sauces is so small compared to when I used to eat a whole piece of bread or bun, it doesn't make me crave more. And, I don't have sauces and gravies every day either.

Sometimes, I will just make cheese sauce with butter, cream, and cheese.

For me, it is keeping the balance of variety, and not getting bored which brings with it the risk of going back to my all-out carb addiction again.

I find boredom in a diet means something needs to change or it is not sustainable.

Pinterest is a great online place to search for Keto, AIP and LCHF recipes.

My Pinterest board is called **Keto and Intermittent Fasting** and has over 200 pins I have found for Keto and AIP recipes.

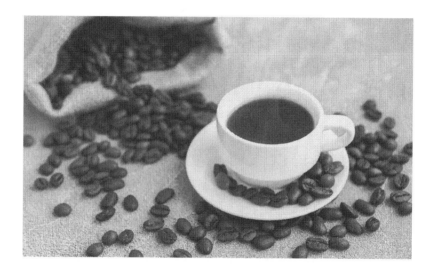

WHAT ABOUT COFFEE, TEA, AND ALCOHOL?

When I started eating low carb, I stopped ordering that "double-double" coffee at the drive-through.

I had never been a big coffee drinker (I typically would have insomnia from the caffeine), but I have enjoyed having it a bit more often now. It is a treat!

I add some unsweetened home-made whipping cream with vanilla. Sometimes I will add some cinnamon to the whipping cream. I'm getting used to no sugar in the coffee and it's still a refreshing drink in the morning.

The same goes for tea. I don't put honey or sugar in my tea now.

When I go to a pub or restaurant, I order mint tea or sparkling water since I don't like the taste of the 0-carb beer.

Beer, wine and cocktails all have some carbs so I try to avoid them in order to not gain back the weight and deal with the issue of insulin resistance.

Making small changes and remembering to have other non-beverage "bridges" can help us get over the challenges of kicking the carb-addiction.

Imagine tasting coffee and tea and not feeling the need to add sugar? This was my experience.

We CAN reset our tastebuds and beat the carb addiction and dependence on sugar.

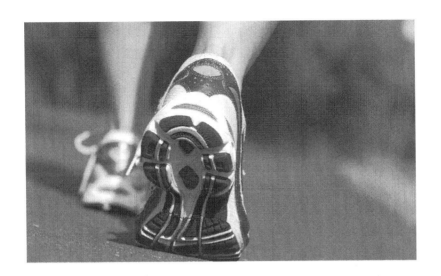

18 - EXERCISE AND FITNESS

WHAT ABOUT EXERCISE AS A WAY TO LOSE WEIGHT?

Most diet and weight loss books will talk about calories in, calories out…needing to exercise to lose weight or exercising to "work off" and justify the food we overeat.

In the past, I have tried to combine starting a diet and starting to get in shape and it never worked well.

Making any big changes in our lives takes will power, self-discipline, planning, and changing our mindsets and habits.

For me, doing something as monumental as losing 80 lbs and adjusting my way of eating was a very big challenge.

I realized I needed to focus on changing what I ate first, and then I could focus on getting my body in shape.

During 2021, I did go for walks, use free weights a few times week, and even went mountain biking and kayaking a couple times but that was near the end of my weight loss.

From what I have been learning, we can't exercise-away a bad diet...we can't out-run our dinner plate.

To put it very simply, if we don't eat, we die. But if we don't exercise, we deteriorate but don't die.

What we put in our mouth – what we eat and when we eat - is the most important thing to focus on.

When I see the progress and success I have had with losing the weight, it motivates me to tackle the next challenge... getting in shape.

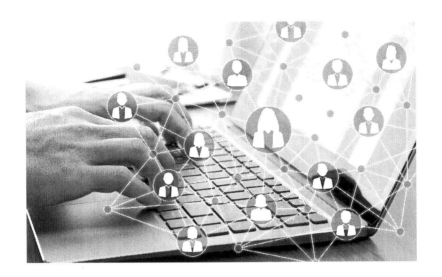

19 - ONLINE COMMUNITY

HOW DO I FIND A SUPPORT GROUP?

Joining an online community helps tremendously with the big learning curve of this new way of eating and fasting.

We are a species that thrive in community. When members of the community evolve, it shows what is possible.

I have been so fortunate to be part of several communities on Facebook that helped me through my most challenging months of getting my health (and body) back.

These groups were so supportive. Some groups even encouraged posting before and after pictures and the response was always so encouraging.

When my hair was falling out from losing weight, I asked the group their recommendation, did what many had advised, and my hair started to grow back fuller than ever.

Each time I came across an obstacle or challenge, I would search the groups and find posts on that topic and 50-100+ people's experiences. I would read about what worked for them and implement some of the changes and find results too.

I was glad I could also help encourage others and make comments on their posts to help them in their weight loss and health journeys as well.

Remember it is OK for us to:

- Ask for help
- Find a support group
- Admit we may be a carb-addict
- Take a long time to achieve our goals if we are moving in the right direction
- Show our "before, during and after" pictures
- Be proud of our results

Here's to all of us who are still evolving, together!

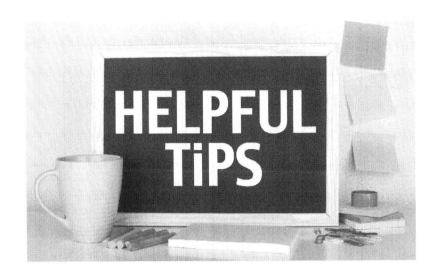

20 - TIPS AND IDEAS

WHAT ARE SOME MORE TIPS TO HELP ME LOSE WEIGHT?

Here are some other tips and ideas that helped me with my weight loss success. These helped keep me motivated and accountable.

JOURNALING

On my phone, I have a notes app. This became my journal. Then I could track how I was feeling, things that I noticed were changing in my daily life, and goals I had for after I had lost the weight.

REASONS WHY

It helped to write a list of all the things I wanted to heal from, health issues and possible future health problems. I put the list on my bedroom wall. By making it obvious, it was hard to avoid and helped keep me accountable to myself.

Even when I felt like I had plateaued, or was not losing weight very fast, I kept the list on the wall. I was not going to let a small slip-up or set-back make me stop.

KEEP TRACK

I purchased 3 inexpensive small notebooks for the following categories:

1. **Carb content** - I made a list of foods to eat and their carb content (only needed this in the first month of going low carb)

2. **Personal Cookbook** - I created a new, personal cookbook by writing out my favourite Keto, AIP, or other low carb recipes. I did this more at the beginning and then used Pinterest later on.

3. **Daily Food Intake** - I wrote down all the foods I ate each day (I did this for the first month of going low carb, till I got the hang of it)

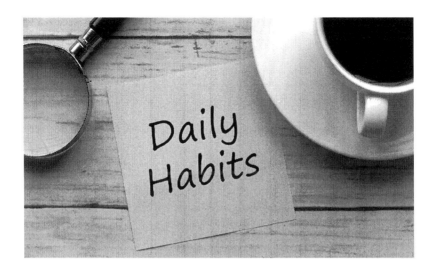

INTERMITTENT FASTING SCHEDULE

There are many free mobile apps to help keep track of intermittent fasting schedule. I used the free version an app and kept track of my fasting and eating windows. There was also an option to keep track of how much water I drank (I used this app for the first 3 months of intermittent fasting).

WEIGHT LOSS TRACKING

I kept track of my weight loss on a piece of paper taped to my bedroom wall. When I weighed myself every day, I would enter that info, every day until I got to my goal weight. Also, I used a weight loss tracking app and I only entered my weekly totals.

MEASUREMENTS

Once every week or two, I would take my measurements. This helped me see how my body was changing. I used a piece of paper on my wall but there are apps for this too. My waist and hip measurements were the ones I kept track of. Those were the most important ones to show I was losing weight.

KEEP LEARNING

By having the goal of learning something new every day, it helped keep the momentum towards recovery. I saved the links to my favourite YouTube videos or podcasts on a mobile app. I'm glad I kept those links since it helped when I was compiling all the references for this book.

OUT OF SIGHT...

One of the most successful things I did near the beginning of going low carb was taking all the high carb/processed foods out of my kitchen cupboards. I stashed them up high, out of reach and in my storage room.

Some of them I gave away and some are still sitting there but I will eventually throw them out. I must admit it's still hard to throw the food in the garbage that I used to eat, and paid money for! But now it's at least out of reach, and out of sight and not tempting me.

TAKE PICTURES

Taking "before" pictures was worth the embarrassment and self-consciousness it caused me. I knew if I did reach my goal, I wanted to remember what I looked like. This is one way to celebrate the "non-scale" victories down the road.

The weigh scale does not show having a smaller double chin, thinner arms, smaller waist, etc. I also took "during" pictures to show my progress.

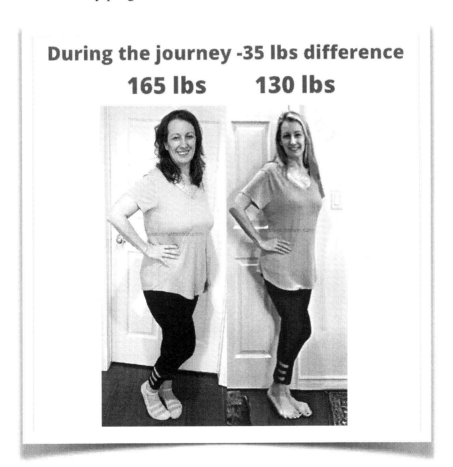

During the journey -35 lbs difference
165 lbs   130 lbs

When I took the "after" photos, I found this very exciting. Once I tried my "fat clothes" on again, I could feel them fitting looser. I needed to gather the cloth at the back to show my profile.

And of course, when I reached my weight loss goal, I took the "after" pictures. I didn't recognize my former self!

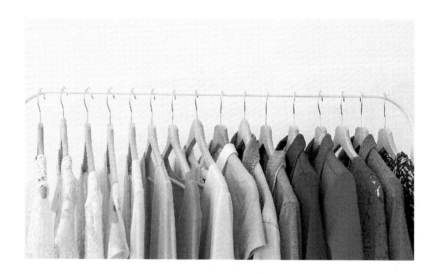

WHAT DO I DO WITH MY FAT CLOTHES?

I am so glad I didn't throw out my "fat clothes" so that I could take the "before", "during" and "after" pictures…to remind myself how far I had come.

While I was obese, I had basically only shopped at the second-hand stores.

As I started losing the weight, it was good to go back and see that instead of needing an XXXL size, I started fitting in XXL, then XL and eventually L, M and S.

Then, I found a store at the local mall that sold new clothes from a previous season at a greatly reduced price and bought some new clothes.

My daughter went through her wardrobe and gave me some things she did not want any more…and now she could borrow from me as well!

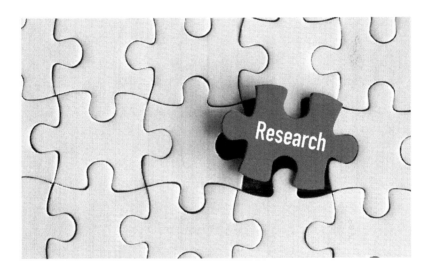

How do you find good medical advice?

NOTE: Just a reminder to read my disclaimer section at the start of this book, if you haven't already done so.

I have found that I cannot always rely on my doctor, dietician, cardiologist, neurologist, therapist etc. to give me the best advice.

Ironically, as I was losing the weight, I noticed the family doctor I had at the time was gaining weight!

Unfortunately, he did not give very good advice. I needed to seek out other doctors and find out what they recommended.

In general, most doctors won't agree with going LCHF, AIP or intermittent fasting since it flies in the face of conventional medicine and the common food pyramids.

It is frustrating when there are new scientific studies and thousands of anecdotal stories showing that there are effective ways to lose weight. Yet it will probably not be told to us by our doctors.

Doing my own research and not listening to only one doctor was the best thing I could do for my health. I did not trust someone who went to university 20, 30, 40 years ago unless they were also keeping up with recent studies and scientific research as well.

For example…

1. If I had only listened to my cardiologist, I would never have done my own research and figured out how to go on the AIP diet, heal my gut and solve my heart palpitations issues.

2. If I had only listened to the neurologist after my mini stroke who told me not exercise very much, I would not have found a 2nd (and 3rd, etc.) opinion which said I should be exercising in spite of my ASD.

3. If I had only listened to my dietician who told me to go on blood pressure medicine instead of losing weight, I would have not solved my high blood pressure issue by losing the weight.

By watching, reading, and listening to others (including the doctors and researchers I mention in this book), I was able to find solutions and healthier options.

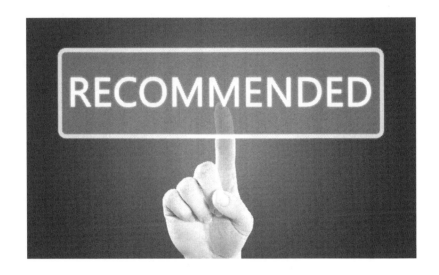

WHERE CAN I FIND MORE RESOURCES?

If you have not already done so, my most recommended resources are in the previous chapters, which I encourage you to review first.

I know there are many books on subjects such as intermittent fasting and LCHF diets.

Since I am an audio and visual learner, I preferred listening to audio books, watching interviews, or listening to podcasts.

Here are a few more recommended interviews, videos, and podcasts that really helped me to find success on this weight loss journey.

INTERVIEWS

Use These Fasting Secrets To Lose Weight & Prevent Cancer! | Jason Fung & Lewis Howes
https://youtu.be/vWg0oBFRZPI

Dr. Robert Cywes personal weight-loss story
https://www.youtube.com/watch?v=hMhj1wmqTiY

Dr Berry Live With Dr Jason Fung; The Cancer Code
https://youtu.be/TiMHLqg1ing

Sugar Addiction; 2 Doctors Discuss
https://www.youtube.com/watch?v=M8Jy8vBN6pk

VIDEOS

Are You A Door Opener? Developing Effective Emotional Strategies Dr. Cywes
https://youtu.be/aaW6XlxjX2Y

Understanding Cholesterol and Statins - Dr. Cywes
https://youtu.be/4leOaX-w89s

Dr. Jason Fung - 'The Aetiology of Obesity'
https://youtu.be/ZKC3hiyLeRc

Best Weight Loss Plans Reviewed (2021) | Jason Fung

https://youtu.be/tYejiLUF0G0

This Causes Cancer! - Fix This To Prevent Disease... | Dr. Jason Fung

https://youtu.be/nrqXKf3tprE

Fat Fiction - Trailer

https://www.youtube.com/watch?v=XzTOBoKOAWA

PODCAST

Diet Doctor Podcast with Dr. Bret Scher - #19 – Dr. Robert Cywes

https://pca.st/episode/1568d1ab-c74c-49b2-bb2a-767a957c9ea6

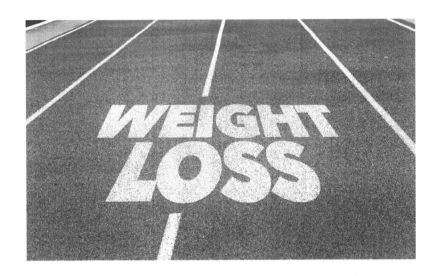

21 - IN CONCLUSION

Losing weight is a marathon, not a sprint!

I hope, if you are overweight or obese like I was, that you take your health seriously...unlike my mistake of ignoring the signs for too long, to my own detriment.

At the time of writing this book, I still have a ways to go to get in better shape. It's a slow process, just like the weight loss was a slow process.

Every day is a challenge to not succumb and go back to my substance addiction (carbs).

It takes mental work, motivation, accountability, daily new habits, and support groups...all the things that people with other substance addictions must have in place too.

It gets simpler but not necessarily easier as time passes... every day making choices for my present and future self.

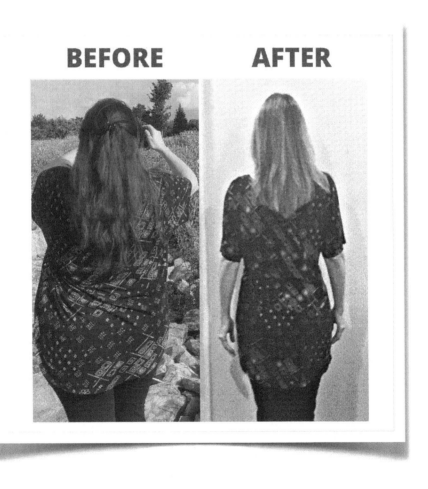

I am in recovery from my carb addiction but also know it could only take 1 day, 1 piece of bread, 1 cinnamon bun, 1 muffin, 1 donut, 1 cookie, or even just 1 bowl of pasta and I might slide back into my addiction again.

I must stay vigilant since I have a history of insulin resistance and can gain weight with very little carbs. My body is having to change from the inside. For me, it is a chemical addiction in that my brain goes crazy when it has carbs, especially grain-based ones.

The carbs turn to sugar and then my body needs more to avoid a "sugar low"...and that cycle repeats.

I remind myself that carbs crave more carbs.

When I don't give my body carbs and feed it with real foods instead (protein and veggies and healthy fat), then it gets fuel from fat and not sugar.

Standing in the candy isle at the grocery store, re-imagining the taste of chocolate, or walking by the bakery dept and smelling fresh bread, it's like a rush to my brain.

I remember tastes, memories of decades of sweet breakfasts, snacks, and desserts.

But now I have a new reality. Here are few examples:

- Wearing size 6 pants
- Wearing size medium 2-piece bathing suits
- Playing frisbee at the beach
- Walking without aches and pains
- Exercising without embarrassment

It was worth the hard work, the DAILY WORK of taking care of this body I have.

I know I am so very LUCKY that my body has recovered, bounced back from being obese.

Yes, there is some loose skin and muscles to tone but I'm getting there...getting to like this body more and more each day...I covered it up for too long.

I choose to either endure my body which will deteriorate faster as I age, if I feed it "bad" carbs and sugar.

Or, I choose to stay away from the sugar and carbs while enjoying the benefits of better health.

It's a freedom to feel in good health and yet the freedom has a daily cost.

It involves sacrificing the huge variety of foods that are out there and choosing only ones that will fuel my body.

Food is literally fuel -
plain and simple.

Now, I must remind
myself to eat. I almost
never get hungry now that
I eat low carb.

My family and friends
have helped so much in
holding me accountable
and yes, occasionally
giving me "ONLY ONE
BITE OF CAKE" and then
taking the fork away!

I couldn't stay in recovery
without all their help. I am
grateful to them.

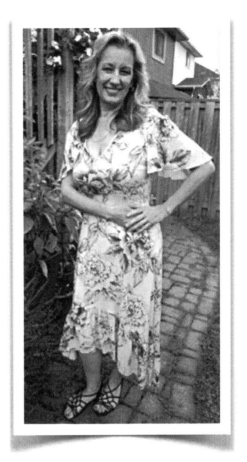

There is so much to gain and it's worth it!!

Do not be afraid to tell your story too (even if you doubt if your words are worth sharing).

People like me were helped tremendously by other people telling their stories.

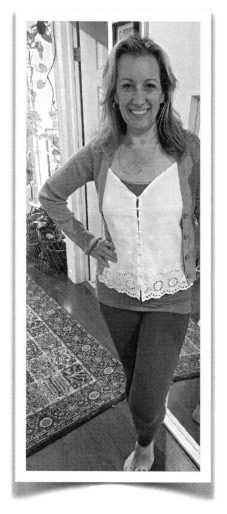

The more we share with each other, the more hope we can pass on to those still struggling.

I am honoured that you chose to read my book and hear about my weight loss success journey.

I would love to hear from you if my story resonated with you and helped you towards your own goal of better health, weight loss and vitality.

You can contact me at:

https://wendynicholson.com/weight-loss-success

REFERENCES

1. "Atrial Septal Defect (ASD)." *Mayo Clinic*, Mayo Foundation for Medical Education and Research, 20 Dec. 2019, https://www.mayoclinic.org/diseases-conditions/atrial-septal-defect/symptoms-causes/syc-20369715#:~:text=An%20atrial%20septal%20defect%20.

2. "Body Dysmorphic Disorder." *Mayo Clinic*, Mayo Foundation for Medical Education and Research, 29 Oct. 2019, https://www.mayoclinic.org/diseases-conditions/body-dysmorphic-disorder/symptoms-causes/syc-20353938.

3. *Bulimia nervosa*. National Eating Disorders Association. (2018, February 22). Retrieved January 13, 2022, from https://www.nationaleatingdisorders.org/learn/by-eating-disorder/bulimia

4. CBNnewsonline. (2016, February 1). *Leaky gut got you down? how to reverse autoimmune disease*. YouTube. Retrieved January 14, 2022, from https://www.youtube.com/watch?v=hk9z4P8kLQ8

5. CrossFitHQ. (2020, July 13). *Interview with dr. Jason Fung and Gary Taubes*. YouTube. Retrieved January 14, 2022, from https://www.youtube.com/watch?v=QAim7IASsEg

6. *Diet 101: Gaps Diet*. Food Network. (n.d.). Retrieved January 16, 2022, from https://www.foodnetwork.com/healthyeats/diets/2019/05/what-is-the-gaps-diet

7. Dr. Andreas Eenfeldt, MD, and MD Dr. Bret Scher. "A Ketogenic Diet for Beginners: The #1 Keto Guide." *Diet Doctor*, Diet Doctor, 14 Dec. 2021, https://www.dietdoctor.com/low-carb/keto.

8. drjasonfung. (2016, March 15). *Fasting and weight loss - solving the two-compartment problem*. YouTube. Retrieved January 14, 2022, from https://www.youtube.com/watch?v=ETkwZIi3R7w

9. drjasonfung. (2020, December 6). *Fasting vs. cutting calories? (the scientific advantage) | Jason Fung*. YouTube. Retrieved January 14, 2022, from https://www.youtube.com/watch?v=5hVX0Aot92k

10. drjasonfung. (2020, December 13). *The physiology of intermittent fasting (science) | Jason Fung*. YouTube. Retrieved January 14, 2022, from https://www.youtube.com/watch?v=DzFpMpi58mY

11. drjasonfung. (2020, December 20). *Intermittent fasting: FAD or future? | Jason Fung*. YouTube. Retrieved January 14, 2022, from https://www.youtube.com/watch?v=CrsqleXWa6Y

12. drjasonfung. (2021, March 7). *Beginning fasting (what to expect) | Jason Fung*. YouTube. Retrieved January 16, 2022, from https://www.youtube.com/watch?v=k8AkF9_hLow&t=14s

13. *Dr. Jason Fung - 'a new paradigm of insulin resistance'*. YouTube. (2017, May 26). Retrieved January 14, 2022, from https://youtu.be/eUiSCEBGxXk

14. equestrain4eva. (2020, October 10). *Intermittent fasting dr Jason Fung [5 stages of fasting]*. YouTube. Retrieved January 14, 2022, from https://www.youtube.com/watch?v=mSOMvC7JHik

15. equestrain4eva. (2021, March 11). *Dr Jason Fung [benefits of longer fasts]*. YouTube. Retrieved January 14, 2022, from https://www.youtube.com/watch?v=KFCyHcDWAn0

16. Fields, L. (2020, April 2). *Atkins diet plan review: Foods, benefits, and risks*. WebMD. Retrieved January 14, 2022, from https://www.webmd.com/diet/a-z/atkins-diet-what-it-is

17. Fields, L. (2021, February 18). *The weigh down diet review: Praying to lose weight?* WebMD. Retrieved January 14, 2022, from https://www.webmd.com/diet/a-z/weigh-down-diet

18. gillianmckeithTV. (2010, May 6). *Gillian MCKEITH: You are what you eat.* YouTube. Retrieved January 13, 2022, from https://www.youtube.com/watch?v=5fkV42JkeIY

19. Maureen Callahan, M. S. (n.d.). *Fit for life.* Health.com. Retrieved January 14, 2022, from https://www.health.com/weight-loss/fit-for-life

20. Mayo Foundation for Medical Education and Research. (2018, February 20). *Anorexia nervosa.* Mayo Clinic. Retrieved January 13, 2022, from https://www.mayoclinic.org/diseases-conditions/anorexia-nervosa/symptoms-causes/syc-20353591

21. Mayo Foundation for Medical Education and Research. (n.d.). *BMI and waist circumference calculator.* Mayo Clinic. Retrieved January 14, 2022, from https://www.mayoclinic.org/diseases-conditions/obesity/in-depth/bmi-calculator/itt-20084938

22. Mayo Foundation for Medical Education and Research. (2020, May 7). *Diverticulitis*. Mayo Clinic. Retrieved January 13, 2022, from https://www.mayoclinic.org/ diseases-conditions/diverticulitis/symptoms-causes/ syc-20371758

23. *Insulin resistance – hormonal obesity VIII*. The Fasting Method. (2014, February 10). Retrieved January 13, 2022, from https://blog.thefastingmethod.com/insulin-resistance-hormonal-obesity-viii/

24. Orenstein, B. W., Lawler, M., Mastroianni, B., Levey, D. K., Migala, J., Fritz, A. L., & Contributor, E. H. G. (n.d.). *Paleo diet 101: Beginner's guide to what to eat and how it works*. EverydayHealth.com. Retrieved January 14, 2022, from https://www.everydayhealth.com/diet-nutrition/the-paleo-diet.aspx

25. *Orthorexia*. National Eating Disorders Association. (2019, December 13). Retrieved January 11, 2022, from https://www.nationaleatingdisorders.org/learn/by-eating-disorder/other/orthorexia

26. Paoli, A., Rubini, A., Volek, J. S., & Grimaldi, K. A. (2013, August). *Beyond weight loss: A review of the therapeutic uses of very-low-carbohydrate (ketogenic) diets*. European journal of clinical nutrition. Retrieved January 16, 2022, from https://www.ncbi.nlm.nih.gov/pmc/articles/PMC3826507/

27. Pathak, Neha. "What Is the Autoimmune Protocol Diet?" *WebMD*, WebMD, 7 July 2021, https://www.webmd.com/diet/autoimmune-protocol-diet#1.

28. Rahmanan, A. (2021, December 14). *Weight Watchers Review*. Forbes. Retrieved January 14, 2022, from https://www.forbes.com/health/body/weight-watchers-review/

29. *The cancer code with dr. Jason Fung – diet doctor podcast*. YouTube. (2021, January 26). Retrieved January 14, 2022, from https://youtu.be/a5ekDT7bScQ

30. "The Great Carbohydrate Debate – How to Lose Weight VIII." *The Fasting Method*, 31 Aug. 2021, https://blog.thefastingmethod.com/the-great-carbohydrate-debate-how-to-lose-weight-viii/.

31. *The sad consequences of the standard american diet*. Atkins. (n.d.). Retrieved January 13, 2022, from https://www.atkins.ca/how-it-works/library/articles/the-sad-consequences-of-the-standard-american-diet

32. "The Science of Intermittent Fasting." *The Fasting Method*, 31 Aug. 2021, https://blog.thefastingmethod.com/the-science-of-intermittent-fasting/.

33. *Tia (transient ischemic attack)*. www.stroke.org. (n.d.). Retrieved January 13, 2022, from https://www.stroke.org/en/about-stroke/types-of-stroke/tia-transient-ischemic-attack

34. *Top autophagy benefits (weight loss)*. The Fasting Method. (2021, July 19). Retrieved January 11, 2022, from https://blog.thefastingmethod.com/top-autophagy-benefits-weight-loss/

35. UCtelevision. (2009, July 30). *Sugar: The bitter truth*. YouTube. Retrieved January 13, 2022, from https://www.youtube.com/watch?v=dBnniua6-oM

36. "What Exactly Is ARFID?" *National Eating Disorders Association*, 20 Feb. 2018, https://www.nationaleatingdisorders.org/blog/what-exactly-arfid.

37. wheatbelly. (2017, July 6). *Wheat belly: Avoid these 7 common mistakes*. YouTube. Retrieved January 14, 2022, from https://www.youtube.com/watch?v=pV-wbEEYcS4

38. ultrawellness. (2020, December 2). *Is cancer caused by Sugar?* YouTube. Retrieved January 14, 2022, from https://www.youtube.com/watch?v=UgUdBEXqE8E

39. YouTube. (2019, January 25). *LCUSA - WPB 2019 - final session*. YouTube. Retrieved January 16, 2022, from https://www.youtube.com/watch?v=wAxReoCNY8c

40. YouTube. (2019, October 29). *EP:04 snacks vs bridges*. YouTube. Retrieved January 13, 2022, from https://www.youtube.com/watch?v=gMmitIkvn5Q

41. YouTube. (2019, December 17). *EP:16 ketogenic rules for: Drinking and hydration*. YouTube. Retrieved January 14, 2022, from https://www.youtube.com/watch?v=XRLC-1QMxOY

42. YouTube. (2020, January 2). *EP:21 Ketogenic Rules for: A healthy liver*. YouTube. Retrieved January 14, 2022, from https://www.youtube.com/watch?v=bJhaUjmgCQQ

43. YouTube. (2020, February 14). *Addiction explained by the carb addiction doc - dr. Rob Cywes*. YouTube. Retrieved January 14, 2022, from https://www.youtube.com/watch?v=_KvBxN5oidc

44. YouTube. (2021, January 28). EP:130 what you must know about yourself before you start keto or recover from a relapse - R. cywes. YouTube. Retrieved January 14, 2022, from https://www.youtube.com/watch?v=XQhjyIrYBSg

45. YouTube. (2021, April 6). *EP:148 when should we eat on a keto diet? Mindblow Time - by Robert Cywes*. YouTube. Retrieved January 14, 2022, from https://www.youtube.com/watch?v=pFjl1S4g2Vw

46. YouTube. (n.d.). *Eating disorders explained: Anorexia, bulimia, Ednos binge.* YouTube. Retrieved January 16, 2022, from https://www.youtube.com/playlist?list=PLAB41960D35357E06

Made in the USA
Columbia, SC
23 July 2024

38992388R00111